WORK

IT

OUT

AVERY

A MEMBER OF PENGUIN PUTNAM INC.

NEW YORK

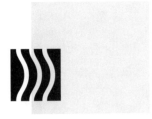

WORK

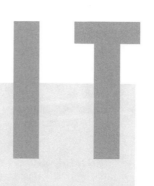
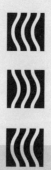

THE BLACK WOMAN'S GUIDE TO
GETTING THE BODY YOU ALWAYS WANTED

IT

MaDonna Grimes

with Jim Rosenthal

OUT

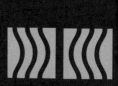

Most Avery books are available at special quantity discounts for bulk purchase for sales promotions, premiums, fund-raising, and educational needs. Special books or book excerpts also can be created to fit specific needs. For details, write Putnam Special Markets, 375 Hudson Street, New York, NY 10014.

a member of
Penguin Putnam Inc.
375 Hudson Street
New York, NY 10014
www.penguinputnam.com

Copyright © 2003 by MaDonna Grimes and Jim Rosenthal
Front cover photograph and first 8-count dance photographs copyright
© 2002 by Robert Reiff & MagicLight Productions, Inc.
Additional 8-count dance photographs (pages 22–29, 31–44, 46–53)
copyright © Scott Ashton. Exercise photographs and "After" photographs on
pages 124 and 125 copyright © Terry Goodlad. Chapter opener photographs
copyright © Kelsey Edwards.

Library of Congress Cataloging-in-Publication Data

Grimes, MaDonna.
Work it out : the black woman's guide to getting the body
you always wanted / MaDonna Grimes with Jim Rosenthal.
p. cm.
Includes index.
ISBN 1-58333-149-2 (alk. paper)
1. Exercise for women—United States.   2. African American women—
Health and hygiene.   I. Rosenthal, Jim.   II. Title.
GV482.G75   2003   2002038473
613.7'045—dc21

Printed in the United States of America
1   3   5   7   9   10   8   6   4   2

This book is printed on acid-free paper. ∞

BOOK DESIGN BY MEIGHAN CAVANAUGH

I would like to dedicate this book to my mom—Evelyn—and grandmother—Genola.

Without them, there would be no me . . .

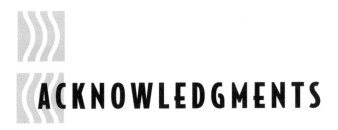

ACKNOWLEDGMENTS

I'd like to thank the following people:

Nikita Grimes, Brigitte Harris-Grimes, Kelvin Grimes, Tony Grimes, Carmen Grimes, Troy Markel, Barry Joyce, Kejo Thomas, Anita Fulgham, Henry Anderson, Michael Waynes, Hazeline Johnson, Yasuyo Honjo, Atsuko Harada, Takako Inamori, Samuel Diaz, Tony Gonzalez, Trevon Hopson, Eugenia Huang, Dan Slick, Jarbé, Tony Stone, Patty Palese, Scott Cole, Sayonarra Motta, Marco Vellegaz, Sally Sagosta, Veronica Durham, Keisha Davis, Beverly Simmons, Irene Rubinsky, Dario Rubinsky, Karen Voight, Henry Seigel, Angel Banos, Stella DeBlik, Anita DeCembly, Jullian Thorne, Judine Rashad Hawkins, Michael Moore, Augustine Rodriguez, Teresa Rodriguez, Eric Pierce, Terrence Pender, Darla and Bill Henry, Matt Terry, Teresa Taylor, Will and Maosa Moore, Bill DeLaney, Mina Ortega, Richard Pacale, Dennis and Sandy Portario, Calvin Whiley, Amy Weinstein, Shelby Henderson, Jeff Dickey, Patrick Goudeau, Marvin A. Smith, Michelle Nevidomsky, Chris Galen, Dr. David Klein, Robert Reif, Fabio and William, Silvana Tucciaroné, Waldo Hernandez, Karen Brodkin, Scott Ashton, Pamela Wright, Sabrina Cochran, Le'Mour Chapman, Tammie Garner, John Peters, Carmen Electra, Marvin Thornton, Frank Williams, Daina Koren, Barry Youngblood, Renee Naja King, Guillermo Gonzalez Vega.

And thanks for all of the support from all of my students across the world.

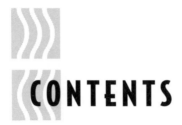

CONTENTS

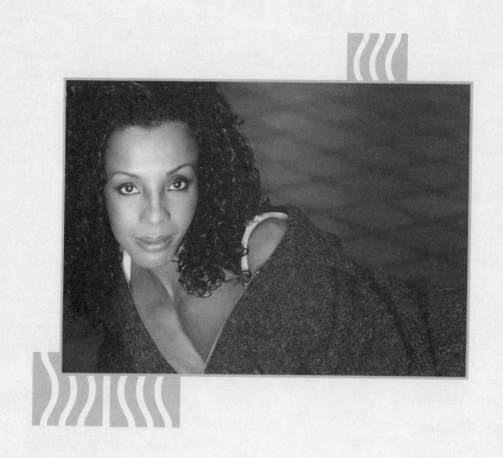

1

Dancing and All That Jazz: An Introduction

I've heard it time and time again—slowly but surely over the years, the pounds just creep on. It was no big deal at first; in fact, you liked your newfound curves, but after a while, you realized that it was time to lose a few pounds. While you knew what you had to do, it was hard to find inspiration. You've picked up weight-loss book after weight-loss book, but they just didn't speak to you. They asked you to do impossible exercises you have no intention of doing, they offer boring meal plans, they have pictures of women on the covers whom you *know* you'll never look like.

Black women have different body types than women of other ethnicities. And no matter how hard we try, we are not going to get our butts to look like the "cute" little ones in the pictures. But why try? African-American women are truly blessed. We have round bottoms and shapely muscles. Embrace those curves that define our heritage. Make time to cultivate your physical, mental, and spiritual dimensions. You have to find the time to figure out what will make you happy and healthy.

This is why I wrote *Work It Out*. I just got tired of watching women with beautiful, shapely curves hold themselves up to impossible "ideals" and try to redesign their bodies into shapes that they were just never meant to be, leaving them feeling like failures in the end. You know how good you can look. Enhance your curves; don't lose them.

And on the other side of the coin are the women who think that they're just fine the way they are. It seems that black women have a very healthy self-esteem, which is great—until it starts affecting your health. Black women disproportionately suffer from obesity. In fact, black women have the highest obesity rate in the country—37.4 percent of us are obese (weighing more than 20 percent above the recommended weight), according to the American Obesity Association Fact Sheet *Obesity in Minority Populations*. Not just over-weight—obese! And while it's wonderful that many women do not let their weight get them down or affect the way they feel about themselves, being overweight is just unhealthy. Obesity is right up there among the top risk factors for diabetes, high blood pressure, cardio-vascular problems like heart attack and stroke, and even cancer. Unfortunately, all of these disorders are far too common among black women.

According to the National Center for Health Statistics, hypertension is most prevalent in the black population, and the rate of hypertension among black women twenty years of age and over from 1988 to 1994 was 35.9 percent compared to 19.7 percent for white women (source: Centers for Disease Control and Prevention, National Center for Health Statistics, Division of Health Examination Statistics).

According to the National Center for Chronic Disease Prevention and Health Promo-tion, in 1999 statistics showed that the prevalence of diabetes (per 100 subjects) in white females ages forty-five to sixty-four was 6.43, compared to 15.52 for black women in the same age group.

According to the American Obesity Association, the obesity rate for black women (37.4 percent) was the highest of any minority group (1998), and the high prevalence of obesity and obesity-related health conditions such as hypertension and type 2 diabetes is a factor contributing to the high death rate from coronary artery disease.

While I'm sure you still look good when you go out at night and turn more than enough heads when you walk down the street, you've gotta make a change for your good health, girl.

That is the gift I am giving you in this special book. In *Work It Out*, I offer you a sim-ple plan to allow you to be consistent when it comes to building and maintaining your body in the years to come. By following my program, you will drop those extra pounds. Then you will show off that new body by toning it. Dieting alone won't do it. I know most sisters, when they see that they're putting on a few extra pounds, decide it's time to go on a diet. I hate to say it, but you gotta work to get the body you want. Not only do you have to exercise aerobically (which will actually be fun with my program), but you've gotta do some weight lifting as well. I can hear the groans already, but once you start seeing results, you'll be hooked. There's nothing sexier than a sculpted body. You'll see. My combination of exercise and diet will radically transform your body. You will change your whole approach toward exercise and food. And these improvements are not temporary. They are designed to last the rest of your life. This is a healthy, *permanent* weight-loss plan.

Most of us turn to weight training and cardiovascular exercise to shed fat and increase our lean body mass. What's less obvious—but even more important—is the connection between exercise and the prevention of diseases prevalent among women. Osteoporosis—a loss of bone mass followed by an increased risk of fracture—is becoming more common in younger women because of a disregard for eating well and getting the right type of exercise.

According to researchers at the National Osteoporosis Foundation in Washington, D.C., the following nine exercises are the most successful in preventing or combating osteoporosis:

- Weight training
- Dancing
- Low-impact aerobics
- Downhill and cross-country skiing
- Walking
- Hiking
- Walking or running on treadmills
- Jogging
- Stair climbing

In my *Work It Out* system, we are integrating dance—a weight-bearing activity that increases skeletal mass—and weight training—a resistance exercise that enhances bone mineralization. Either way, you are increasing blood flow to your bones and helping to prevent osteoporosis.

I have put together a system of training to motivate and inspire you to work it out and get in shape. I'm not talking about just going to the gym three or four times per week. I'm talking about adding dance—hip-hop, African, and Latin styles are the ones I specialize in—to the workout mix.

I provide you with some basic dance exercises that you can do at home, but it's also good to mix it up by taking some aerobic dance classes. It will take time to find the appropriate dance classes in your neighborhood, but they are out there for the taking. Use weight training to stay toned and cardio to stabilize your metabolism—now your life is almost complete.

Changing your life is easier than you think. Here is my approach to life:

Food = Fuel

Exercise = Energy

Simply changing your relationship with food and exercise can make all the difference in the world.

I eat enough food to give me energy to complete my day. I know when to stop eating a meal because my body tells me when I'm full. I eat only when hungry. If I'm in a social situation, I will snack on fruit or salad.

As I get older, the need to exercise becomes even more pressing. I rely on my fitness regimen to relieve stress, give me more energy, and experience more joy. When you exercise, the feeling is pure joy—you are more in touch with your body and your soul.

It is so important to read through each chapter and understand the importance of incorporating every part of the program into your busy schedule. Stretching and flexibility exercises can be performed in the comfort and privacy of your home. The abdominal circuit can be performed before going to work or before going to bed. I'm going to give you the information, but it is up to you to find the time to make it happen.

Bless you and good luck!

THE MADONNA GRIMES STORY

Life has been good to me. I can't tell you how amazing it is to be able to earn my living as a dancer and hip-hop instructor who has worked with such headline performers as LL Cool J, Pink, Destiny's Child, and MC Hammer and to have traveled the world teaching hip-hop workshops—my special gift that has brought so much pleasure and satisfaction.

Everywhere I travel, the questions always get around to my body: specifically, what it is that I'm doing to stay in shape all the time. The connection between dance and exercise is very clear: Constant movement (dance) burns calories and builds endurance and mind-body awareness. The best part of the process is that dancing is fun. It is a natural expression of culture, love for music, and getting in touch with the physical, and sensual expression of who and what we are as black women.

My love for dance goes back to my childhood in Knoxville, Tennessee, and Dayton, Ohio. I never took dance classes, as my parents were working hard just to get by. But I got my education in the street-dance talent shows that were—and still are—so popular in the South and Midwest.

I hung out with about fifteen other kids, and we formed a dance group known as the Enchanters—a crew of eight-year-old boys and girls doing slickly choreographed routines in the streets of Dayton. I won my first contest when I was eleven—handing it to those older girls and showing them how it was done—and started to enter talent shows all over town. Soon, I was collaborating with many of the best young dancers, and we started winning disco dance contests at clubs to earn some money.

When I was eight years old I was lucky enough to move with my parents to Dayton, Ohio, where I went to high school, joined the cheerleading squad, competed in gymnastics, and was exposed to a diverse cultural, social, and racial environment. I never lacked confidence in my ability—no matter what I put my mind to I had a way of doing well, and so during my senior year in high school I auditioned for the dance department at Ohio State University in Columbus—a huge campus with more than fifty thousand students. I was a small-town girl but totally into the challenge of putting my dance talent on the line in front of the faculty of one of the best dance programs in the United States.

I did not have one day of formal dance training in an actual "school" but auditioned in both modern and ballet and was accepted to OSU for the following fall semester, where I majored in dance and theater. The dance faculty thought it was kind of funny that I had no technical background in dance, but they were willing to give me an opportunity, and for that I'll always be grateful.

The one thing that saved me from starving for four years was a spur-of-the-moment decision to go out for the cheerleading team. I was just barely getting by on food stamps during my freshman year; I was lucky if I had enough money to eat one meal per day. I went to an open tryout that I heard about from friends in the dance department, and those other girls did not stand a chance. I was doing toe jumps and back handsprings and dance moves—stuff that no one else had even seen before. The OSU athletic department gave me a scholarship assistance, and my days of starving were finally over.

While at OSU, I did a lot of the dance choreography for the cheerleading team, and our squad was one of the top schools in the country. I became so tight with the cheerleading program that years after leaving school, I still went back to campus to choreograph the routines for the NCAA National Cheerleading Championship competitions.

I went straight from Ohio State to the center of the dance universe—New York City, of course—and was accepted into the master's program in dance choreography at New York University. I was always ambitious and never satisfied with doing just one thing at a time. And so I immediately went to the Dance Theater of Harlem's Summer Program in dance and auditioned for and got a job as a dancer in the Broadway production of *Bubblin' Brown Sugar*.

My Broadway credits from that period include *Jesus Christ Superstar, Cats,* and *Sesame Street Live*. No matter how busy I was as a professional dancer, I somehow managed to keep up with my work at NYU—don't ask me how I was able to do it—and ultimately graduated with my masters in choreography performance.

And even though my life was full with school and dance performances, I let some of my cheerleading friends talk me into competing in the National Aerobics Championships. Remember that this was a big deal back in those days—it was televised on NBC TV and sponsored by Crystal Light. Athletes were flown into L.A. from all over the world (including a girl named MaDonna!). I won the National Aerobics Championships on my very first try, flew back to NYC to return to Broadway and NYU, and—strangely enough—started getting requests from the other aerobics competitors to choreograph their routines.

Now, I was being paid to travel to Brazil to teach hip-hop workshops. I pretty much invented the class with a hybrid style of jazz and hip-hop; all I really did was apply my craft as a dancer to aerobics, and it was a big-time success.

The touring continued, and it was all kind of crazy and exciting. I was making regular coast-to-coast trips to Los Angeles to work with several top-level aerobic champions. And when I had a short break in my schedule (a rarity, to the say the least), I took a job performing in a musical production and coordinating fitness on a cruise ship.

I did not have a clue about the ins and outs of strength training or teaching aerobics for the purpose of getting in shape or losing weight, but I was lucky enough and resourceful enough to figure it out on my own. Thanks to the money I was able to save from that one job, I was finally in a position financially to move to L.A. and start my dance and acting career for real.

THE DANCE-FITNESS CONNECTION

My dance-workout program took shape in the early '90s in a West Hollywood dance studio called Voight Fitness. I had been taking classes there for several months, and many of the other students wanted me to teach a class.

I did not really have a set plan. My goal was just to go with my groove. And Voight Fitness put a hip-hop dance series together based on my system. They heavily promoted the classes, and because of that buzz, my very first class was packed with dancers. I invented the name Cardio Hip-Hop because my students expected to be able to burn calories and get lean through dance — and that's exactly what I'm going to teach you how to do.

After two years of leading jam-packed classes at Voight, I decided to get on with my life and make something happen. I started devising plans with my friend Irene Rubinsky to open up our own dance studio. We saved barely enough cash to open the school — it was one big room (what passed for a studio) and a very small rehearsal space. The odds were stacked against us from day one, but word of mouth got out to the dance community, and dancers from all over the world started flying in to take my classes.

I was one of the first dance teachers to integrate cardio and hip-hop into a program of exercise that's fun, motivational, and a terrific workout. I divided my class into sections that you will follow in the dance phase of the Work It Out program:

The Warm-up: ten to fifteen minutes of light movement, including walking and arm movements.

The Stretch: two minutes of some basic stretches to enhance total-body flexibility.

Cardio: This part consists of constant dance movements without resting — just moving from one dance to the next without stopping, as if you are letting it fly on the dance floor of a club.

The Routine: The dance movements become more structured and are blended into a routine to improve endurance, conditioning, and flexibility while integrating the dance moves into an actual cardio workout.

The Cooldown: Finish with a circuit of crunches and other various midsection exercises to strengthen and tone the core—the abdominals, lower back, and trunk.

Since devising this system, I have opened my own dance studio, competed in and won professional fitness contests, and done magazine shoots for fitness and fashion magazines, including *Glamour* and *Allure*.

Almost every sister I meet asks me how I got "the body," with abs and a tight butt and muscle tone that's feminine and appealing. The answer is pretty basic: I never miss a day of working out.

You can do it, too. And the best part is that you'll have fun and nonstop pleasure as you see major changes in how you look and feel—inside and out.

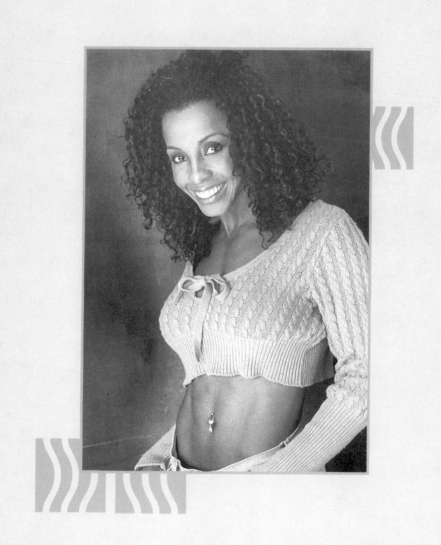

2

Get into the Groove:
The Fat-Burning Dance Workout

Sisters can relate to the beauty and poetry of human movement and the many pleasures of listening to music and moving to the beat.

I have always loved dancing since I was a little girl. It makes me happy and energized. It can change my mood from depressed to excited and optimistic. And best of all, dancing is an effective method of burning calories and getting into shape. I know a lot of sisters—too many of them—who don't like to "work out." Dance is a fun alternative to conventional workouts. It's a lot of fun, and it's easy to forget that you're working out. I also know a lot of sisters—an awful lot—who love to do their thing on the dance floor. They didn't realize that if they did it long enough and consistently enough, that it could serve as a workout.

My plan is simple: We are going to start with a three-day-per-week dance program that you can do at home until you start taking classes at a local studio. Let's set aside Tuesday, Thursday, and Saturday for dancing; and Monday, Wednesday, and Friday will be your strength and cardio days.

There's no limit to the number of dance styles that will get your heart racing and your body moving, but we're going to begin with three styles that I enjoy teaching and performing: *Afro-Latino*, *Dance Street*, and *Cardio Dance*.

THE BENEFITS OF THE DANCE/FITNESS PROGRAM

I'm going to get you hooked on dance, and after that it will become an important part of your social life and regular routine. You'll make lots of cool friends in dance class. It is a party atmosphere, where you sweat like crazy. Dance classes enable you to burn more calories than any other physical activity, with the exception of running or cycling, and my hip-hop drills will keep you limber, flexible, and coordinated.

Dance—which teaches you how to move your feet, arms, and legs quickly—is an athletic skill that transfers easily to many other recreational sports. Now you'll be used to moving your body in many different directions. And dance is an effective method of training both fast-twitch muscles—the muscle cells that fire quickly (anaerobic)—and slow-twitch muscles—muscles that contract slowly (aerobic or endurance).

My friends tell me that I'd be great at kickboxing, surfing, or in-line skating because my dance training has taught me so much about balance, coordination, and flexibility. But I'm a rabbit of habit when it comes to sweating: I go with the one physical activity that always gives me pleasure and stimulation. And that means I'm a dancer, pure and simple.

Dance class keeps you moving faster and looking and feeling younger than any other workout class. Many women learn to train with weights and do cardiovascular exercise, but when you combine those methods of getting into shape with dancing you have a triple threat that is unbeatable.

And—this is my favorite part: Your sex life will improve once you start to dance. Dance teaches you more about how to move your body around in all sorts of exciting positions. Flexibility, elasticity, and endurance all blend together in a very sexy way. Sex is a big part of your life, sister, and I'm promising a better way to go at it thanks to this program.

GETTING STARTED

The photos and dance styles in this chapter will get you plugged in to a consistent three-day-per-week dance/workout schedule. I'll get to the specifics in a minute or two. But once you are hooked on dancing, you should start taking classes at a local dance studio or health club. If you live in a big city like New York or Los Angeles, you can find these cardio/dance classes in studios; for everyone else, though, the best bet is to check out local health clubs for classes that keep you moving.

Hip-hop and funk are very popular. But you have to put in the time to investigate the options to find types of music and teachers who inspire you. I travel all over the United States and always manage to locate classes that work for me.

Think of this book as an opportunity to take my class. We're going to hang out together, sweat together, and get motivated to stay in shape together. I'll keep everything moving, shake things up, and make sure you stay focused on being consistent from start to finish.

Now, keep in mind that as you're following my directions, I want you to *mirror* my moves. So, since you're facing "me" (this book), and I'm facing you, your left will be my right. Nonetheless, I will still move on the side corresponding to the side I want *you* to move. For instance, if I say, "Lift your left foot," in the accompanying picture my right foot will be lifted because I am facing you and want you to mirror my action. This is the proper way to teach dance technique. You'll get the hang of it once you get started.

CALCULATING A TARGET HEART RATE

Before you begin, you must determine your target heart rate—just how much you should safely get your heart working during your workouts. Burning fat and training correctly require some important background information. Being aware of your target and maximum heart rates will help you train efficiently and minimize the chances of overtraining.

These are the four easy steps to calculating your target heart rate:

1. First you must determine your resting heart rate: Relax. Check your pulse rate for ten seconds and multiply that number by 6. The product is your resting heart rate, which you can use as a reference point. The lower the resting heart rate, the higher the target heart range.
2. Estimate your maximum heart rate by subtracting your age from 220. This number is your max heart rate.
3. Select an appropriate target zone. Most doctors and exercise professionals recommend a target range of 55 to 85 percent of your max heart rate. As you'd

expect, the higher the percentage, the more intense the workout. Never exceed 85 percent, though.

4. Determine your target heart-training range with this formula:

To make this easy, we'll say you are a forty-year-old who wants to train at 60 percent of her max heart rate.

$$220 - 40 = 180 \text{ (maximum heart rate)}$$
$$180 \times .60 = 108 \text{ (target heart range)}$$

THE WARM-UP

Slip into comfortable clothing and throw on some music to get you going. Pick a tune that has tons of energy. Janet Jackson, Michael Jackson, and Britney Spears are three of my favorite warm-up choices.

My goal is to make you break into a sweat and warm up your body. Walk around the room to the music. Jump around. Move from side to side. Don't think—just move it! Throw on some music and party for about 10 minutes.

THE STRETCH

Do standing lunges (without weights) to stretch quads, hamstrings, and hips. See page 68 in chapter 3 for photos of this exercise if you're not entirely sure how to do it. Bend your lead knee to stretch the thigh, then extend the front leg to stretch the hamstrings. Repeat the stretch on both legs. And repeat 10 times.

Follow with a standing stretch for the lower back. Spread your legs apart (what is known as "second position") and bend your knees (or plié) about halfway down with hands on your thighs. Inhale to push abdominals in; exhale to push abdominals out to arch your back; repeat 10 times.

Also, drop your head to your shoulder and move your head from side to side to stretch the neck muscles. Do head circles. Move hips from side to side, forward and back, (10 reps per stretch) and you are ready to begin the routine.

TUESDAY: DANCE STREET

This is a street-dance style integrated with jazz, which means plenty of turns. The clothes I'm wearing in the photos are what's cool in the hip-hop world. And hip-hop is essentially a street dance that goes with a blend of rap and rhythm and blues. Everything is up-tempo and fast. Clothes are flowing, comfortable, and breathable. The attitude is young. But older rappers (thirty-somethings) have a more solid reputation than the younger rappers.

RECOMMENDED MUSIC

Rap: Mr. Cheeks, Lil' Bow Wow, Snoop Dogg, Jay-Z, Ja Rule, Nas. These are just a few examples—go with what you like to dance to. R&B: Michael Jackson's *Invincible* or *Off the Wall*.

WORKOUT FORMAT

I want you to do your dance workouts for thirty consecutive minutes. I'm going to start you off with a few basic eight-count dances to go with different styles of music. Remember that the movements from one step to the next should be fluid. Don't do a step. Stop. Do a step. Stop. Just keep moving. Remember: This is dancing. Just keep moving with the music. Practice the moves for a couple of minutes to get them down before you begin your thirty-minute workout. And these eight-count dances are a basis for your workout. Use them as a starting point but improvise as you go along. Just do what the music tells you to do, as long as you keep it moving. The plan is to have a blast while you're whipping that bod into shape.

Ready? Let's go.

DANCE STREET EIGHT-COUNT #1

COUNTS   1   AND   2

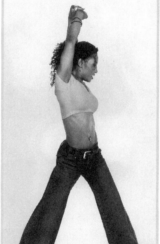
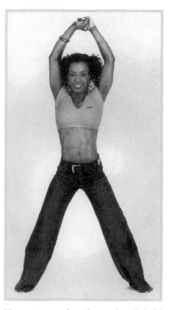

Spread your legs apart (or hop out second, in dance lingo), with your hands held together high overhead.

Twist to the right.

Hop out second, with your hands held together high overhead.

AND

3

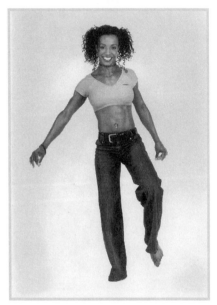

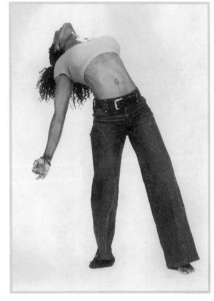

Turn your body to the front position and hop onto your left foot.

"Body roll"—push your knees, hips, stomach, and head out and then back, moving from the bottom to the top of your body.

4   5

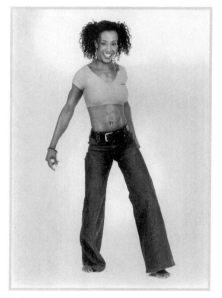

Roll back into a standing position.

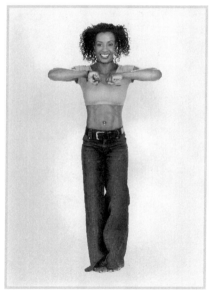

"Hop" to bring your feet together and your arms
to your chest . . .

AND

6

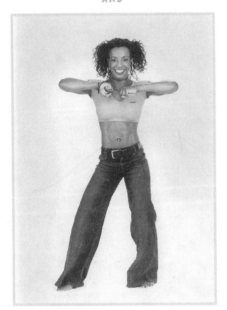

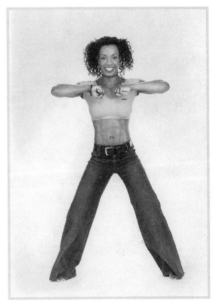

. . . and step to the left.

Step with your right foot to the right to spread your legs just past shoulder width . . .

AND

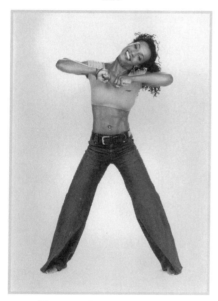

. . . and bring your head to your right shoulder.

7

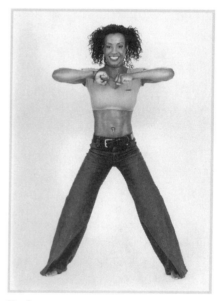

Head up . . .

AND

8

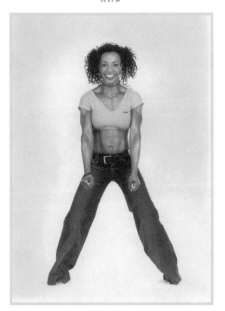

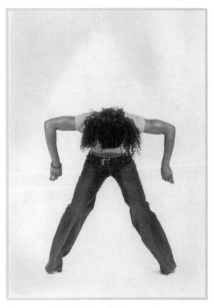

. . . and begin to circle your arms. Begin with arms down toward your legs and circle, bringing them upward over your head.

Arms complete circle—all the way down.

DANCE STREET EIGHT-COUNT #2

COUNTS   1   2, 3

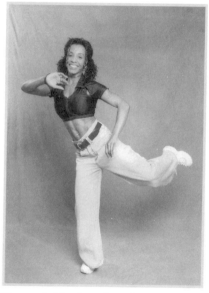

Step your left foot forward and flick your right leg up behind you.

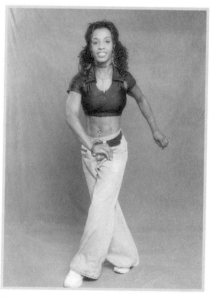

Cross your right foot over the left. Hold this position for the 3 count . . .

AND

4

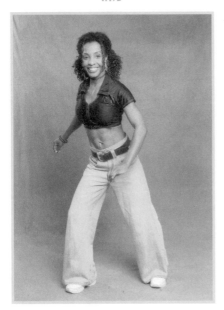

. . . and step to the left.

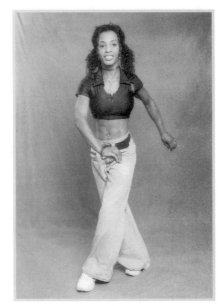

Cross your right foot over the left.

5

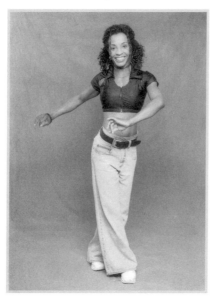

Cross your left foot over the right. Hold this position.

6, 7

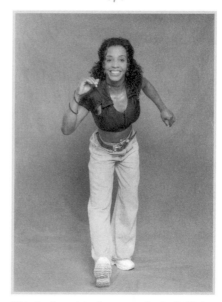

Slide back as right foot moves back. Hold this position . . .

AND

8

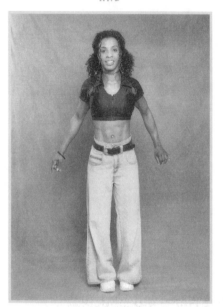

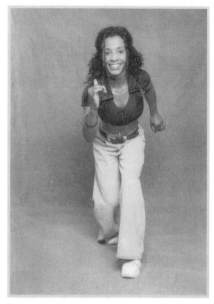

. . . and bring left foot back, parallel to the right foot.

Bring right foot forward.

Dance Street Eight-Count #3

COUNTS   1   2

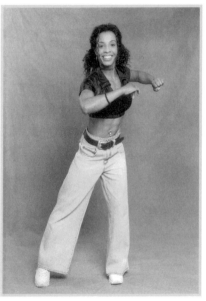

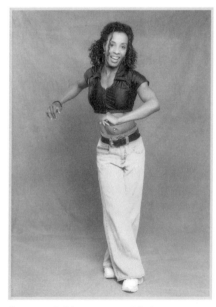

Mambo left—step your left leg and your hips out
to the left.

Cross your left leg over your right leg.

3

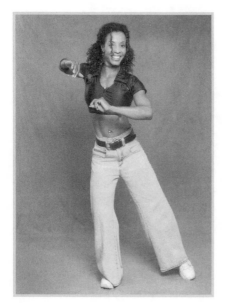

4

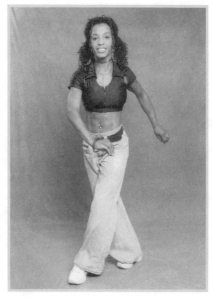

Mambo right—step your right leg and your hips
out to the right.

Cross your right foot over the left.

COUNTS   AND   5   6

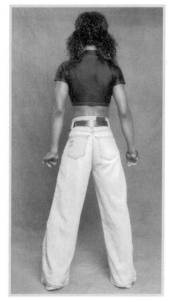 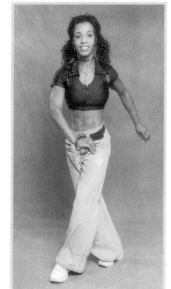 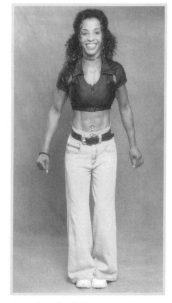

Face back.

Cross your right foot over the left.

Complete the full turn; you are now facing front with your feet together.

7

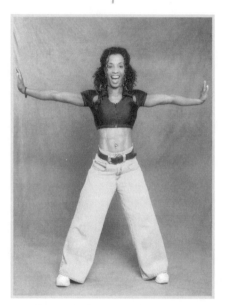

8

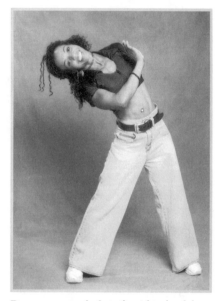

Extend your right foot out wide to the right, arms out to the side.

Drop your upper body to the right—head drops to the right; arms drop right in front (of the body) with left arm in back.

THURSDAY: AFRO-LATINO

This is my synthesis of Latin dances (salsa, mambo, samba from Brazil) and a traditional African dance (the Gang Gang). Try incorporating colorful, exotic, sexy clothes into the workout like the ones I wear in the photos to fully get you into the spirit of the workout. Fun clothes and bright colors are motivational and keep you happy while you're dancing. Put on some lipstick and makeup. Check yourself out in the mirror, and you will like what you see.

RECOMMENDED MUSIC

A mix of African drums and Latin jazz, salsa, and Brazilian samba. The music is much faster than what you'd get in a Dance Street class.

WORKOUT FORMAT

This workout consists of thirty minutes of nonstop dancing with a much faster tempo and more intensity than the Dance Street session. The Afro-Latino eight beat (taken from the traditional African Song—"The Gang Gang Song") gives you a blueprint for choreographing a thirty-minute dance routine that will work for this genre of music.

This is an African dance called the Gang Gang.

AFRO-LATINO EIGHT-COUNT #1

COUNTS   1   2

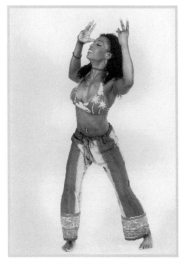

Step to the right with arms at shoulder level bent upward ("with arms"). Lean into the step with your torso twisted a bit to the left.

Step to the left with arms. Lean into the step with your torso twisted a bit to the right.

3 AND 4

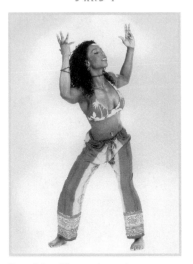

Step right with arms (repeat).

Work It Out

5

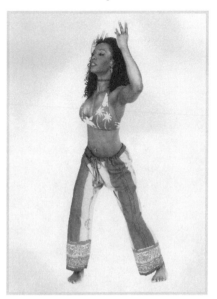

Step left with arms.

6

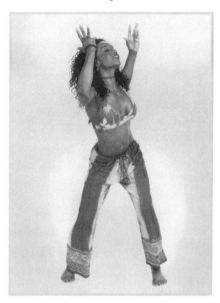

Step right with arms.

7 AND 8

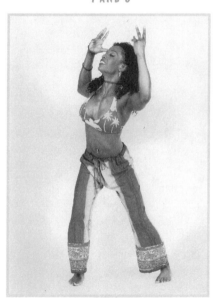

Step left with arms (repeat).

AFRO-LATINO EIGHT-COUNT #2

AND

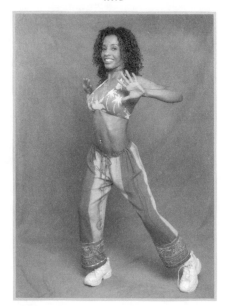

1

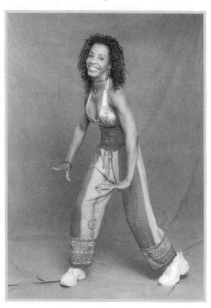

Hop left, facing your upper body to the left, with your back arched, your chest pushed out, and both hands held at mid-chest level (pump position).

Release the pump by pushing your upper body back and your arms down.

AND

2

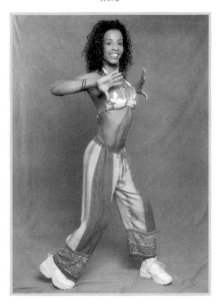 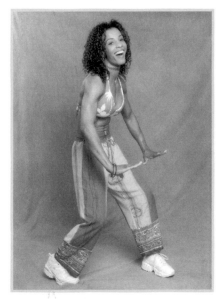

Hop right, facing your upper body to the right, with your back arched, your chest pushed out, and both hands at mid-chest level (pump position).

Release the pump by pushing your upper body back and your arms down.

AND

3

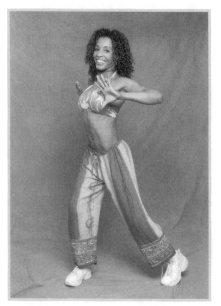

Hop left, facing your upper body to the left, with your back arched, your chest pushed out, and both hands at mid-chest level (pump position).

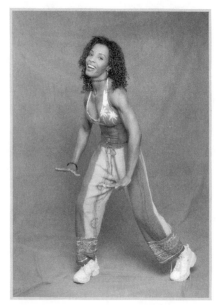

Release the pump by pushing your upper body back and your arms down.

AND

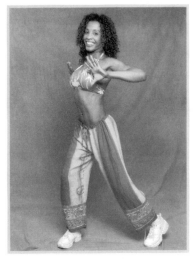

Hop left, facing your upper body to the left, with your back arched, your chest pushed out, and both hands at mid-chest level (pump position).

4

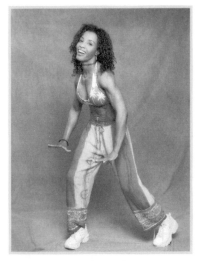

Release the pump by pushing your upper body back and your arms down.

AND

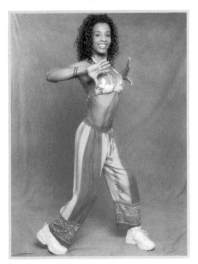

Hop right, facing your upper body to the right, with your back arched, your chest pushed out, and both hands at mid-chest level (pump position).

5

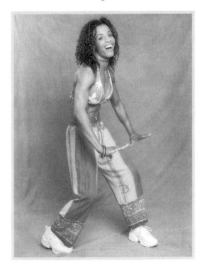

Release the pump by pushing your upper body back and your arms down.

AND

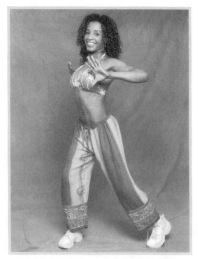

Hop left, facing your upper body to the left, with your back arched, your chest pushed out, and both hands at mid-chest level (pump position).

6

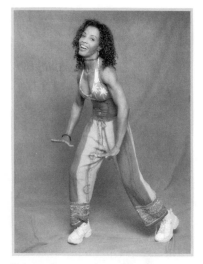

Release the pump by pushing your upper body back and your arms down.

AND

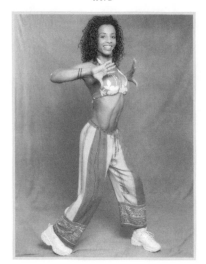

Hop right, facing your upper body to the right, with your back arched, your chest pushed out, and both hands at mid-chest level (pump position).

7

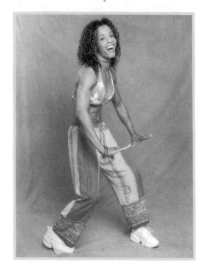

Release the pump by pushing your upper body back and your arms down.

AND

8

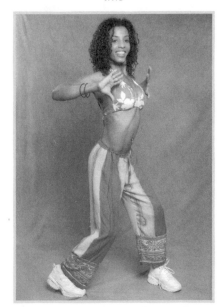

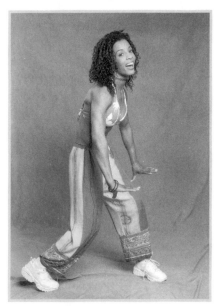

Stay in the same position and repeat the pump—bring both hands to mid-chest level and arch.

Release the pump by pushing your upper body back.

REPEAT.

AFRO-LATINO EIGHT-COUNT #3

1

AND

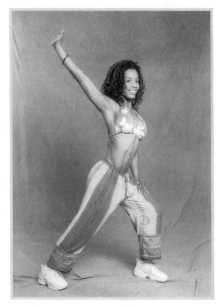

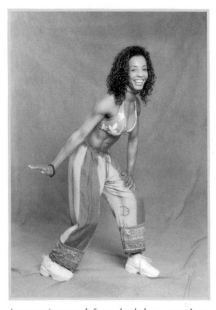

Step back with your left foot and arch your body. Swing your left arm up above your head and to the side.

As you swing your left arm back down, step down with your right foot as you release the arch and bring your hips forward.

2

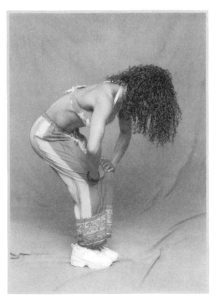

3

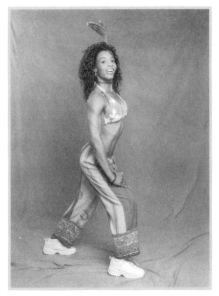

Bring your left foot forward together with your right foot as you make a complete circle with your arms and bend down.

Now, repeat this movement on your other side. Begin by swinging your right arm above your head; take a step back with your right foot and arch.

AND

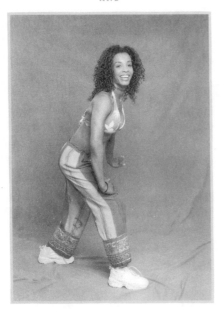

4

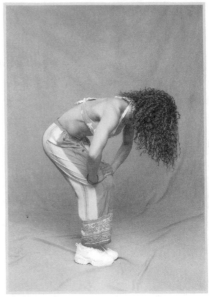

Swing your right arm down and step down with your left foot as you release the arch and thrust your hips forward.

Bring your right foot together with the left foot; make a complete circle with your arms and bend down.

AND

5

AND

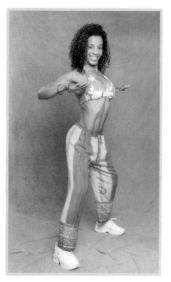

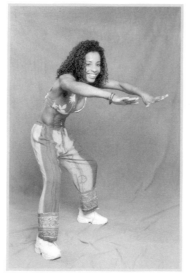

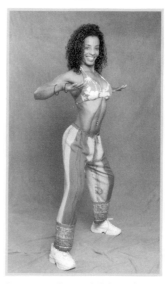

Step out with your left leg, opening your legs wide, with your upper body arched and hands at mid-chest level.

With your arms at chest height, push your upper body back. Then pump again, arching your back. Release the pump by pushing back.

Step out with your left leg, opening your legs wide, with your upper body arched and hands at mid-chest level.

6

AND

7

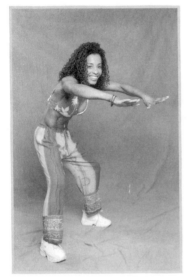

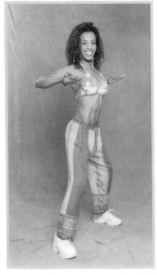

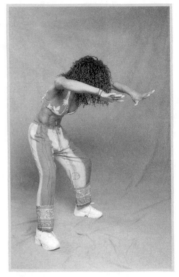

With your arms at chest height, push your upper body back. Then pump again, arching your back. Release the pump by pushing back.

In the same position, arch with hands at chest height.

Then release the pump, pushing your body back, with your head down and your arms extended out in front of you, elbows slightly out to the sides.

AND

8

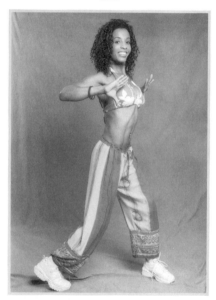

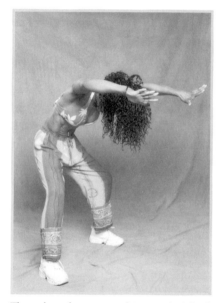

Arch again, bringing your head back to its nor-
mal position and hands back to chest level.

Then release the pump, pushing your body back
as your head bends down and your arms extend
all the way out to the side.

SATURDAY: CARDIO DANCE

This class is very similar to Dance Street. The only difference is that the movement is simpler and it is repeated over and over again. This style is ideal for club dancers who find one basic riff on the dance floor and just go with it all the time. It is for people who do not want to put a lot of little dance elements together in a routine that they are forced to remember. But it is funk, rap, pop, drums, and R&B all mixed together. It's a very generic class because you can get away with almost anything—as long as you are moving constantly.

RECOMMENDED MUSIC

Janet Jackson, Britney Spears, Pink, and Destiny's Child are good choices, as you are repeating the same steps and the goal is to sweat.

WORKOUT FORMAT

I like to get my dancers to take this class because it is all about burning calories and fat. This is the best style for working out because of the simplicity of movement. Dance Street is the hardest style to apply to a workout, as you are moving slower and in a more down-in-the-groove-to-the-rap mode. Not every sister can burn calories to Snoop Dog, but it's well worth the effort. Afro-Latino falls somewhere in the middle, but it is very up-tempo and will keep your heart pumping for thirty minutes.

CARDIO DANCE EIGHT-COUNT #1

COUNTS   1   2

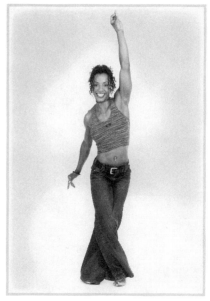 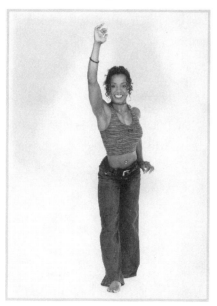

Step with your left leg over your right leg, and punch your right arm up in the air.

Step back to the right, and punch your left arm up in the air.

3

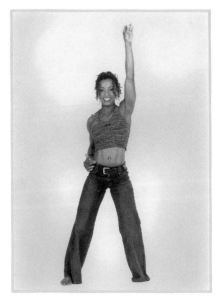

4

Step the left leg out to the left, bringing legs just slightly wider than shoulder width apart, and punch your right arm up in the air.

Step with your right leg over your left leg, and punch your left arm up in the air.

5

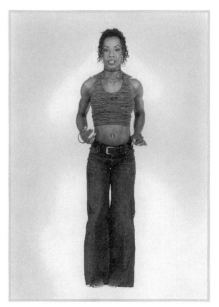

Step to the left side, bringing your legs together, arms at your sides.

6

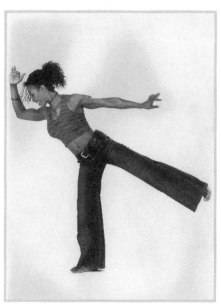

Lean your torso to the left and kick your right leg out in the air.

7

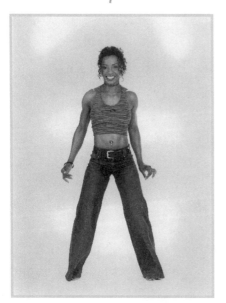

Step to the right, with your arms at your sides.

8

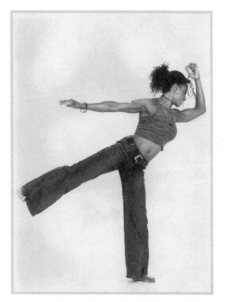

Lean your torso to the right and kick your left leg out in the air.

CARDIO DANCE EIGHT-COUNT #2

1

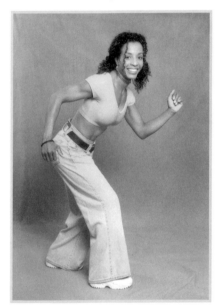

2

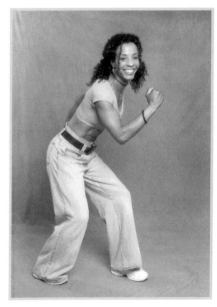

Bending at the waist just a little, step with your left foot to the left.

Step to the right with your left foot, still slightly stooped.

3

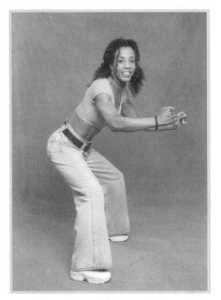

Push your hips back while bending both knees; move your arms forward.

4

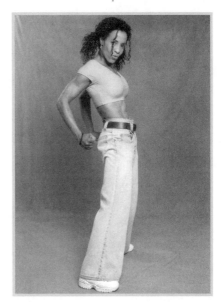

Drive your hips forward with your knees slightly bent. Bring your arms back toward your hips.

5

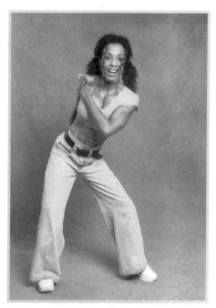

Bending at the waist, step wide to the left and place your right hand on your left shoulder.

6

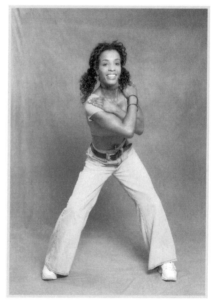

Step to the right and place your left hand on your right shoulder, crossing your arms over your chest.

7

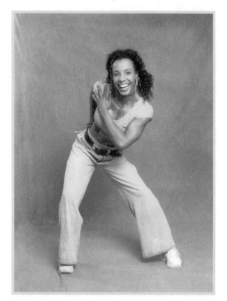

8

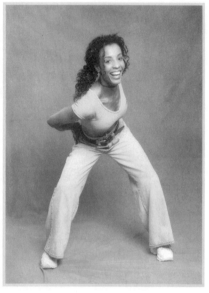

Step to the left, slightly bent over, and put your left hand on your butt.

Step to the right, bend over, and put your right hand on your butt.

GREAT EXPECTATIONS

This is not a short-term workout program designed for only short-term success. It must be accompanied by the weight-training, abs, stretching, and nutrition information that follows in the next three chapters. But I promise you that if you begin to dance three days per week, you will burn fat and change your body very quickly. Most sisters who take dance will drop a dress size in a couple of weeks. Your friends will think you are starving yourself or doing two hours of cardio per day.

Go take a dance class, use my dance-workout program as intended, and you won't need starvation diets and extreme workout programs. My plan is designed for black women in pursuit of a personal-best body for keeps.

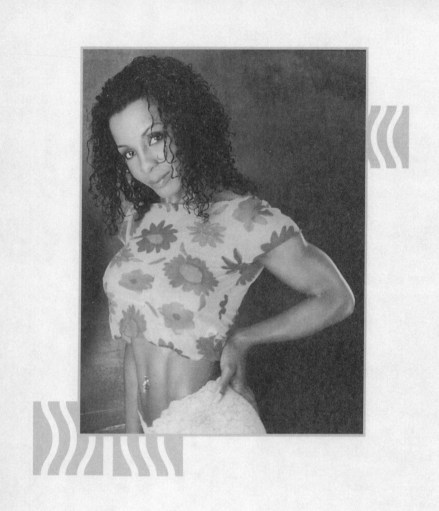

3

Strength Is Beautiful: My Weight-Training and Cardio Clinic for Building a Better Body

Listen, I know that you have special needs. It took me a long time to get into the groove of training. That's no big thing. We all go through funks when hanging out and watching TV seem better than sweating. But once you start experiencing the pleasures of looking better and feeling better, it's easy to get it going on all the time. You have to do your cardio and you have to do your weight training. All I'm asking for is three days each week of your precious time. Forget about a quick-fix solution. I want to set the tone for a lifetime of success, health, and well-being.

We all need role models to inspire and help put us on the right track to making progress. I'm just like you in every way, and I know what you need to prod that body into top shape. Of course, throughout this book you should remember that I've got your back—everything has been tested and retested over my many years of training as a professional dancer, aerobics athlete, and fitness competitor.

ANATOMY 101

One other item of business before starting a weight-training routine is to get down with the street about anatomy: Believe it or not, your beautiful body has over six hundred distinct muscles. For the purpose of limiting this anatomy lesson to what you need to know, we'll subdivide the body into target zones for the weight-training workout you'll be hooking up with in the pages that follow.

QUADRICEPS, HAMSTRINGS, AND GLUTES

The quadriceps are the four muscles at the front of the thigh that extend and straighten the leg. The four muscles are the *rectus femoris*, the *vastus intermedius* (these two create the V-shape of the mid-front thigh), the *vastus medialis* (inner thigh) and *vastus lateralis* (outer thigh). The hamstrings, also known as the leg biceps and located at the back of the upper leg, must be trained with weights for strength and stretched to ensure flexibility when dancing or performing any sport that requires lower body strength or endurance. The glutes are the butt muscles. We all know how hard it is to slim down the glutes and streamline and shape the quadriceps. The plain truth is that the upper thigh muscles are the largest in the entire body and they come into play in almost every sport and physical activity.

ABDOMINALS

Upper and lower abdominals (abs) and obliques (the muscles of the abdomen and waist) are instrumental in building a body that's beautiful, sexy, and strong at the core. Most lower-back problems come from the dreaded combination of weak abs and too much fat around the midsection. A dancer needs a strong, flexible waist and so does any woman who wants a strong, sexy physique.

The *rectus abdominis*, which flexes the spinal column and pulls the sternum toward the pelvis, is the long ab muscle that begins at the pubic bone and inserts into the cartilage of the fifth, sixth, and seventh ribs. The external obliques, used to rotate and flex the spinal column, are the muscles at either side of the torso.

BICEPS

The upper and lower biceps give the arm shape, muscle clarity, and definition. With well-defined biceps, you are sending a message that you are strong and self-confident and have got it going on!

The *biceps brachii*, which curls and lifts the arm, is a two-headed muscle that begins under the shoulder and inserts below the elbow.

TRICEPS

Most women store fat at the back of the upper arm. There's an easy solution to this problem if you are willing to train right: Just tone up those triceps. You'll burn the fat stored there, while defining the muscle.

The *triceps brachii*, which straightens the arm, is a three-headed muscle that (like the biceps) attaches below the elbow and under the shoulder.

THE BACK

With the back, size is not the goal. Definition, shape, and a hint of width are where it's at. The key muscle is the *latissimus dorsi*, which holds the spine upright. The lats—shorthand for the *latissimus dorsi*—pull the shoulder back in rowing exercises and pull the shoulders down in pulldowns or chinning exercises.

SHOULDERS

We are out for shape, separation, and balance among the front, side, and rear heads of the deltoid muscle.

The deltoid, which lifts and rotates the arm, is a three-headed muscle (shaped like a triangle) that begins at the clavicle (collarbone) and inserts in the upper arm.

CHEST

Detailing the chest muscles is priority number one. Toning these muscles will not only make you look great in tank tops and low-cut tops but will also help prevent your breasts from sagging.

The pectoral muscles pull the shoulder and arm across the front of your body. The upper pec is attached to the clavicle; the largest section of the pectorals starts at the upper-arm bone, then fans out to cover the rib cage.

GUIDELINES AND OTHER GOOD STUFF

DRESS FOR COMFORT

I like to wear clothes that are comfortable and practical when working out. Don't worry about buying expensive workout apparel. Go with what feels right to sweat in.

FORM IS THE KEY

I've included detailed explanations of how to perform each exercise in the program. This how-to information along with my anecdotal comments on each exercise is enough to get you started. Never do an exercise before you know how it works. Do not hesitate to ask a more experienced trainer to help you get it right.

WARM UP BEFORE YOU TRAIN

I'm telling you to do thirty minutes of cardiovascular exercise *before* weight training to elevate your heart rate and to get the blood moving into the muscles.

WORK OUT WITH YOUR MIND AS WELL AS YOUR BODY

The mind-muscle connection is one of the most important training principles. It is so simple: Visualize what you want your body to look like as you lift weights; focus your mind on the muscle group you are targeting, not the mechanical up-and-down or side-to-side movement of the dumbbells or handles of a machine.

THE WEIGHT-TRAINING DICTIONARY

Okay, we are almost ready to get this party started. Just a few more things. I'm sure that some of you have lifted weights before—with varying degrees of success—but let's review a few of the most basic (and important) elements of resistance training.

THE REP

A rep is one full cycle of an exercise—a contraction of the muscle followed immediately by an extension (or stretch) of the muscle. A set is a group of any number of repetitions. All workouts are organized into sets and reps. I will tell you how many reps to perform per exercise. Select a weight that will allow you to complete each rep with perfect form.

TRAINING TO FAILURE

This means keeping a set going until you cannot complete any more reps at that given weight without stopping. This is the kind of thing you'll see bodybuilders or more advanced trainers experimenting with, and it is something I want you to avoid. We are using lighter weights and placing emphasis on perfect form.

FULL RANGE OF MOTION

Each lift of the weight should take the muscle from full extension (stretch) to a complete contraction. This method is the only way to trigger results.

RECUPERATION

The basic training in this routine allows for a brief recovery period for the muscles being stimulated through the forces of resistance. Despite what many women believe, progress with the program (definition, shape, and quality of muscle) takes place during periods of recuperation. If you train too often, therefore, overtraining and fatigue prevent any progress.

FREQUENCY

You will train Monday, Wednesday, and Friday without fail. Monday and Friday are set aside for legs and glutes (lower body), as this is the main target zone of the program. Train your upper body on Wednesdays—you can always add a second upper-body workout if a particular body part or muscle group requires special attention.

REST BETWEEN SETS

My system is based on taking minimal (ten to twenty seconds) rest between sets of exercises. The goal is to complete the workout in a minimum amount of time—because I know that you don't have much time to spare—and because the goal is to build lean muscle while also burning fat.

Supersets are two exercises that you perform in a row without stopping. It is even possible to perform three sets in a row (a triset) or four or more exercises in a row (a giant set). Supersets can be organized in two ways: two exercises in succession for the same bodypart or two exercises in succession for two different bodyparts. I will generally superset within the same bodypart, but in my Aerobic Weight Training System on page 79, I will superset triceps (triceps pressdowns) with biceps (dumbbell curls), and dumbbell curls (biceps) with shoulders (shoulder presses and lateral raises).

THE SPLIT

A split routine is a method of mixing and matching muscle groups to maximize progress. Split routines are an efficient way of dividing up the entire body into distinct bodyparts (such as training biceps and triceps together in the same workout) or training zones (such as upper body or lower body). The goal is to prioritize your training while increasing efficiency—getting the most done in the minimum amount of time.

I've split up the three days to focus on the target areas for women's training. Most sisters need to place more attention on the lower body. We've got rounded bottoms that require shaping and sculpting. Our legs always need more quality muscle and definition. Hamstrings offer flexible strength for dance, aerobics, and all endurance sports.

We are blessed with strong, well-developed upper-body muscle groups, and so one day per week is usually okay to get things started.

THE WORK IT OUT WEIGHT-TRAINING PROGRAM

The first step of your weight training is, believe it or not, cardio. You've got to engage in twenty to thirty minutes of some kind of cardio exercise to warm up your muscles. You can go with either the treadmill or the stationary bike; both will burn calories while elevating your heart rate to its target range.

The stationary bike is ideal for women who want to spare their knees and ankles from the wear and tear of the treadmill. Stationary bikes are easy to use and comfortable for most body compositions. And electronic feedback such as target heart rate, calories burned per hour, and an estimate of distance traveled during the workout is also useful for assessing your productivity.

Personally, I love doing my cardio on a treadmill. It works you harder than the bike. You can incline the treadmill to make it even more challenging. And, of course, you get all the same electronic programs for motivation that go with the stationary bike.

Selecting your favorite mode of cardio is a personal matter. I've known women who were in great shape but hated running on the treadmill because it caused pain in the ankles or knees. And I've talked to women who think the bike is too boring. Whatever you decide is cool as long as you pick one or the other and stick with the twenty- to thirty-minute interval, three days per week, every single week.

Step two of the weight-training program is the actual weight training. I'm telling you that this workout should not last more than thirty minutes. What's the point of wasting precious time? I want you in and out of the gym with the best possible outcome for your time invested. Unless I say otherwise for a specific exercise, start with the minimum comfortable weight, and over time as it gets easier to lift that weight, work your way up in 10-pound increments.

Here's a typical leg workout for Monday and Friday. On Wednesday you hit the upper body, and we'll get to that good stuff in a minute. For now, a few comments about each of the exercises you'll be performing.

LEGS/LOWER BODY

Exercise One: Dumbbell Squats—4 Sets of 12 Reps

Start with 20-pound dumbbells and work your way up to heavier weights as you begin to feel stronger and confident in your form. I vary my stance to train different parts of the thigh. A wider (past-shoulder-width) stance shifts the emphasis to the inner thigh and hamstrings. With legs together, I work quads more than hamstrings. Vary stances from one week to the next or stick with one stance you feel most comfortable with and that best suits your goals and priorities.

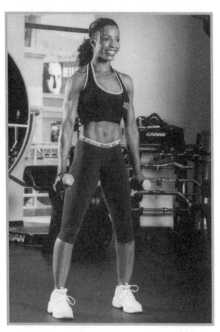 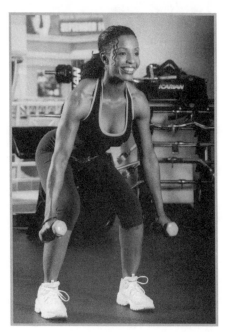

Stand with a dumbbell in either hand, feet spaced shoulder width apart. Keep your head up and back straight. Squat until your thighs are parallel to the floor. Keep your head up. Return to the starting position. Don't lock your hips out at the top of the movement. Don't bend your wrists while lifting the weight.

Exercise Two: Leg Extensions—4 Sets of 15 Reps

The leg-extension machine strengthens your quadriceps to support the integrity of your joints, tendons, and ligaments and to prevent knee injuries. It is a controlled movement—the machine has a predetermined range of motion that keeps you safe and focused on working the muscle. Bring your legs up to a count of 1, 2—pause at the top for a contraction and then lower the weight to a count of 3, 4, before returning to the starting position.

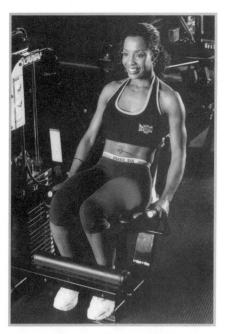 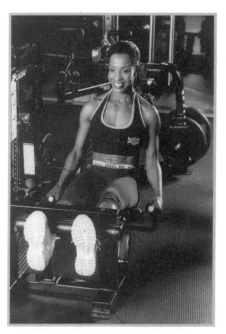

Hook your feet under the pads of a leg extension machine. Extend your legs as far as they'll go until they lock out to achieve a peak contraction—hold for a count of one-two, then lower the weight slowly until your feet are just below your knees (the starting position).

Exercise Three: Leg Curls—4 Sets of 15 Reps

Every gym has a version of a leg-curl machine, and it is the best way to stretch and contract the hamstrings—the muscles at the back of your legs. Strong, flexible hamstrings are essential for injury prevention and the ability to execute the dance moves in chapter 2. Typically, women have put more emphasis on training the front of their thighs than their hamstrings for obvious reasons: You can see your thighs, but you can't see your hamstrings. All muscle groups must be trained equally from front to back.

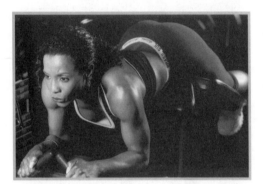 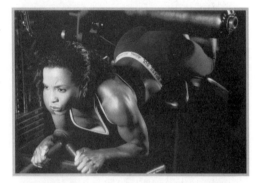

Lie prone on a leg-curl machine and set your heels under the pads of the mechanism. At the outset, your legs are stretched out straight. Hold on to the handles to keep your body from moving. Supporting yourself on your elbows also helps to make sure your body stays firmly on the bench. With your hips tucked and body in a fixed position, curl your legs up as far as your range of motion will allow, contracting your hamstrings—hold for a count of one—at the top of the movement. Slowly release and return to the starting position.

Exercise Four: Dumbbell Lunges——4 Sets of 15 Reps

The cool thing about lunges is that you are blending hamstring, thigh, and glute trainings into one fluid movement. I'm a believer in using dumbbells, (15–20 pounds on average) rather than a barbell, as it is a safer technique—no stress is placed on the spine as you are stepping forward into the lunge position.

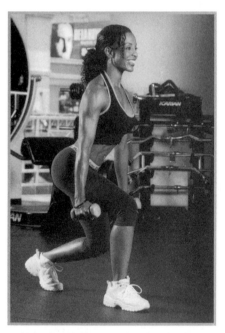 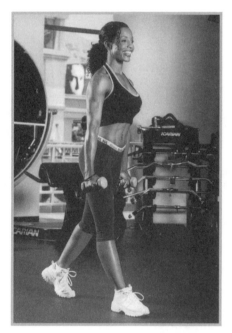

Hold the dumbbells at arm's length, palms facing in. Keep your head up and back straight. Step forward with the right leg until the upper thigh is as close to parallel (to the ground) as possible. Then step back to the starting position and repeat on the other leg. I often perform these as walking lunges, moving one step at a time and alternating legs as I go through a full range of motion and stretch out my thighs and hamstrings.

UPPER BODY

Exercise One: Wide-Grip Pulldowns—2-4 Sets of 10-15 Reps

This movement is similar to a chin-up, but you do not have to rely on your body weight for resistance. Always squeeze your back muscles as you pull the bar down to your neck to take the emphasis off your biceps.

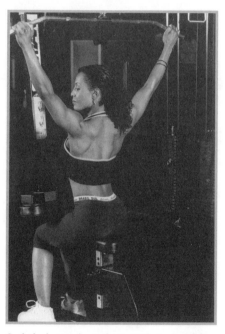
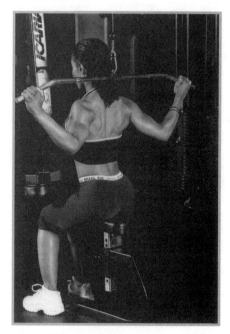

Grab the bars in front of you. Sit facing a pulldown machine with a wide (well past shoulder-width) grip on the bar. With your arms fully extended at the starting position, pull the bar straight down until it touches the back of your neck. Hold for the contraction. Slowly return to the starting position. Rely on the muscles of your upper back, rather than your arms, to handle the resistance of the weight.

Exercise Two: One-Arm Dumbbell Rows—2-4 Sets of 10-15 Reps

I like this exercise for two reasons: It isolates the back muscles on each side of your body and allows you to lift the weights higher to get a more complete contraction.

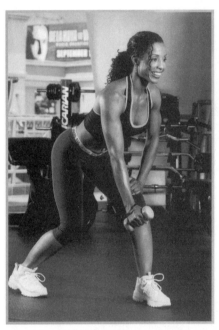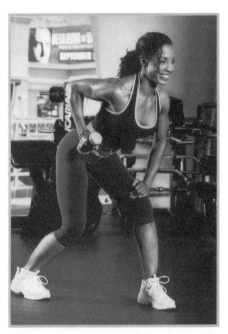

Place a dumbbell in front of you, either on the floor or on a bench. Grasp the dumbbell with your right (working) hand and rest the left hand on your left thigh for support. Begin with the dumbbell at arm's length. Lift the dumbbell straight up to the side of your chest, keeping your arm close to your side. Return to the starting position, retracing the same path. Reverse position and repeat the movement on the left side.

Exercise Three: Dumbbell Flat Bench Presses—2-4 Sets of 10-15 Reps

Using dumbbells rather than barbells or a machine enables you to lift through a more complete range of motion; balancing the weights also trains coordination and endurance.

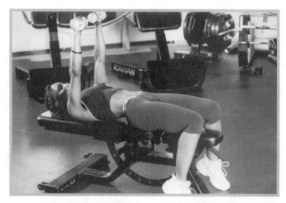

Lie on a flat bench, take a dumbbell in each hand and hold the weights straight overhead with palms facing forward. Lower the weights to the outer chest, keeping them under control at all times. Lower as far as your range of motion will allow, feeling a good stretch in the chest muscles. Press the dumbbells back overhead until the arms are locked out (fully extended) at the top.

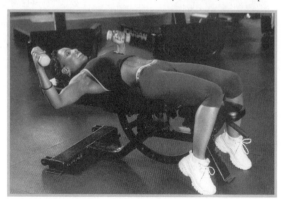

Exercise Four: Incline Dumbbell Flyers—2-4 Sets of 10-15 Reps

With this exercise, you are stretching, detailing, and toning the upper chest, which is the only part of the chest most people will see when you are wearing a bikini at the beach.

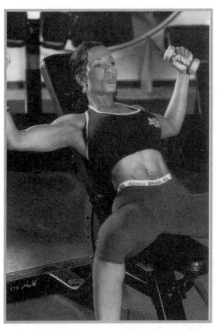 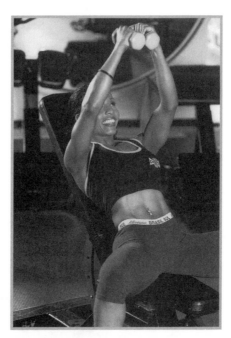

Lie on an incline bench with the dumbbells held straight overhead, palms facing each other. Lower the weights out and down to either side in a wide arc, bending the elbows slightly and keeping the palms facing each other. Lower until the chest gets a full stretch and then retrace the arc to the starting position.

Exercise Five: Triceps Pressdowns—2-3 Sets of 10-15 Reps or Triceps Kickbacks—2-3 sets of 10-15 Reps

Alternate between these two exercises from one upper-body workout to the next. Pressdowns strengthen and build the triceps muscle, while the kickbacks are more of a fine-tuning movement.

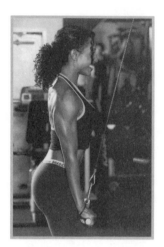 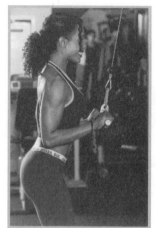

Attach a short bar to an overhead cable and pulley on the triceps-pressdown machine; grasp the bar with a palms-down grip. Make sure your elbows are locked into place and close in to your sides during the entire exercise. Keep your body in a fixed position. Do not lean forward. Begin with your arms parallel to the floor and press the bar down as far as you can, locking out your arms and contracting the triceps at the bottom. Release and slowly bring the bar up to the starting position.

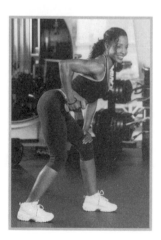 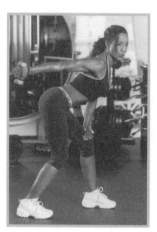

For triceps kickbacks, stand bent at the waist, with your knees bent, left foot in front of the right, with your left hand resting on your front thigh or a low bench for balance and stabilization. Grasp a dumbbell with your right hand. Bend the arm behind you with the dumbbell hanging straight down below the elbow and raise your forearm straight back and up to shoulder height, pressing the weight back until your arm is parallel to the floor. Keep your elbow in close to your side. Hold for one second to squeeze and contract the triceps. Slowly return to the starting position. Complete all your reps on the right arm before repeating the movement with your left arm.

Exercise Six: Standing Dumbbell Curls—2-3 Sets of 10-15 Reps, or Hammer Curls—2-3 Sets of 10-15 Reps

You can flip-flop these two exercises in your upper-body session or go with the movement that is better suited to your training objectives. Dumbbell curls fully contract the biceps to shape the muscle; hammer curls (a variation on standard dumbbell curls where the palms face inward throughout the exercise) shift the emphasis from upper biceps to lower biceps and forearms.

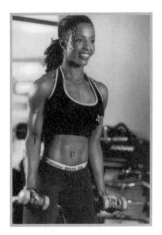 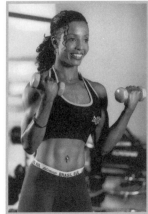

Hold the dumbbells at your sides. Stand up straight. Keeping your elbows steady, curl the dumbbells forward so that the thumbs turn to the outside, with palms facing up. Lift the weights as high as you can while still feeling a contraction in the biceps (for me, that means to shoulder height), and then slowly lower the weights until your arms are hanging down at your sides.

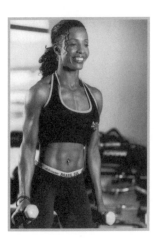 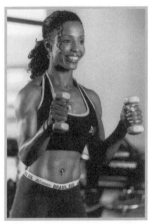

The hammer curls are performed the same way, only the palms face inward throughout the range of motion.

Exercise Seven: Dumbbell Shoulder Presses—2-3 Sets of 10-15 Reps, or Front Raises—2-3 Sets of 10-15 Reps

Each exercise develops the front (anterior) head of the shoulder, which is the part of the deltoid that gets the most resistance when you train your chest or triceps; or lift your arms over your head while you perform many of the dance steps in chapter 2.

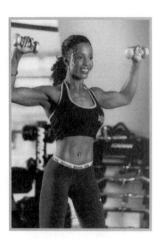 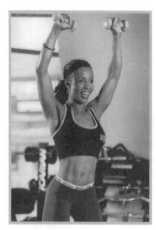

Hold a dumbbell in each hand at shoulder height (or slightly higher as in the photo). Lift the weights straight up until the elbows lock out at the top. Lower to shoulder height (or just above it), and repeat.

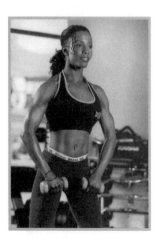 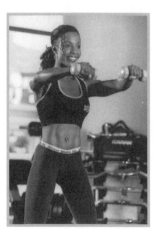

For front raises, stand with a dumbbell in each hand. Lift both dumbbells up out in front of you to shoulder height. Hold for a contraction in the shoulder. Slowly lower to the starting position, and repeat.

Exercise Eight: Standing Lateral Raises—2-3 Sets of 10-12 Reps

Finish with the best exercise for hitting the outer (medial) head of the deltoid. Don't lift the dumbbells too high (above shoulder height) or you will limit the resistance.

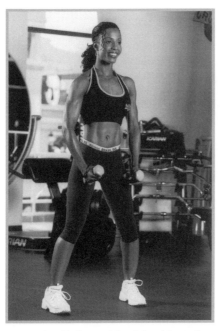
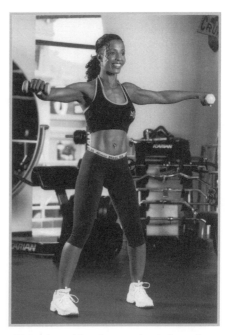

Grasp a dumbbell in each hand, bend forward just a little, and bring the weights close together in front of you. Lift the dumbbells up and out to shoulder height, turning your wrist ever so slightly so that the back of the dumbbell is higher than the front of the dumbbell. Slowly lower the weights to the starting position. Do not swing the dumbbells up and down. Focus on using your shoulder muscles to handle the brunt of the resistance.

MADONNA GRIMES'S STRENGTH-IS-BEAUTIFUL PROGRAM

Workout One*

MONDAY AND FRIDAY

BODY PART	EXERCISE	SETS	REPS
Legs/Glutes	Dumbbell Squats	4	12
Quads	Leg Extensions	4	15
Hamstrings	Leg Curls	4	15
Quads/Hamstrings/Glutes	Dumbbell Lunges	4	15

*Begin with thirty minutes of cardio (either treadmill or stationary bike) at 55 to 85 percent of your max heart rate.

Workout Two*

WEDNESDAY

BODY PART	EXERCISE	SETS	REPS
Back	Wide-Grip Pulldowns	2–4	10–15
Back	One-Arm Dumbbell Rows	10–15	2–4
Chest	Dumbbell Flat Bench Presses	2–4	10–15

*Begin with thirty minutes of cardio (either treadmill or stationary bike) at 55 to 85 percent of your max heart rate.

Workout Two (continued)			
WEDNESDAY			
BODY PART	EXERCISE	SETS	REPS
Chest	Incline Dumbbell Flyers	2–4	10–15
Triceps	Triceps Pressdowns or Triceps Kickbacks	2–3	10–15
Biceps	Standing Dumbbell Curls or Hammer Curls	2–3	10–15
Shoulders	Dumbbell Shoulder Presses or Front Raises	2–3	10–15
Shoulders	Standing Lateral Raises	2–3	10–15

MADONNA GRIMES'S AEROBIC WEIGHT-TRAINING SYSTEM

I've devised an alternative weight-training system that can be used in addition to the primary program or—if you are really looking to lean out—in place of the "Strength is Beautiful" workout.

Lower Body (Monday and Friday)

Do each exercise with no rest in between sets. Once again, we are using the supersetting technique to improve endurance, burn calories, and add sleek muscle tone. Use a very light weight for any exercise requiring dumbbells or machines.

CIRCUIT 1

1 set of leg curls—15 reps, 30 pounds

1 set of leg extensions—15 reps, 30 pounds

1 set of crunches

Repeat this circuit 3 or 4 times.

CIRCUIT 2

1 set of lunges (no weight)

1 set of crunches

1 set of lunges (no weight)

Repeat this circuit 3 or 4 times.

Upper Body (Wednesday)

CIRCUIT 1

1 set of wide-grip pulldowns (10–15 reps)

10 push-ups

1 set of one-arm dumbbell rows (10–15 reps)

Repeat circuit 2–4 times.

CIRCUIT 2

1 set of flat dumbbell bench presses (10–15 reps)

20 crunches

1 set of incline dumbbell flyers (10–15 reps)

Repeat circuit 2–4 times.

CIRCUIT 3

1 set of triceps pressdowns (10–15 reps)

1 set of dumbbell curls (10–15 reps)

20 jumping jacks

1 set of lateral raises (10–15 reps)

1 set of dumbbell shoulder presses (10–15 reps)

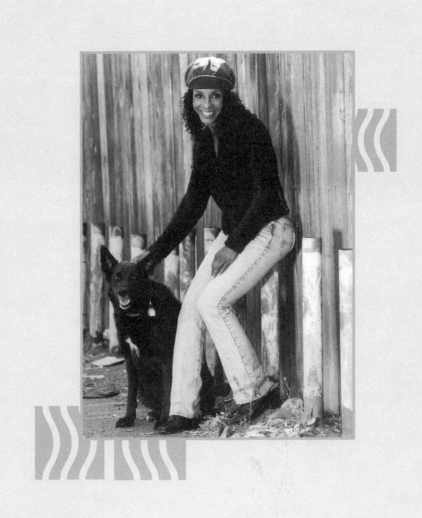

4

Flexible to the Core:
The Abdominal and Stretching Plan

I'm going to make you a promise: In the time it takes to pull into the drive-thru at Jack in the Box and eat a burger and fries and wash it down with a chocolate shake, you can work your abdominals to prevent lower-back and hamstring injuries and stretch every muscle to ward off pulls, strains, and damage to your joints, tendons, and ligaments.

Many of the fitness women I train slack off when it comes to finding time to train their abs and to stretch properly—and they end up paying the price for this neglect by getting injured and missing competitions.

Abdominal training and stretching function as the prevention side of my fitness plan. Hitting the abs six times per week will tone the midsection and strengthen the torso at its core—the core is the centerline at the waist where the lower and upper body come together at the hips and pelvis. The lower-back region (*erector spinae* muscles) is, without a doubt, your weakest link. Toning the abs is the only way to transform that weak link into a strong and functional body part that will hold up when you dance, do your cardio, walk, or perform any type of exercise.

Flexible muscles are required for safe, effective weight training, dancing, and even performing day-to-day movements like bending over to pick up your kids or getting in and out of an automobile. Stretching exercises should (much like abs) be performed six days per week. Both of these programs are unique. Forget about sets and reps and just move continuously from one exercise to another for five to ten minutes. Perform each abdominal exercise for sixty seconds without resting, before immediately moving on to the next exercise in the program.

THE ABDOMINAL SESSION

Perform this program after weight training (Monday, Wednesday, and Friday) and after dance (Tuesday, Thursday, and Saturday) when your body is all warmed up.

Beginners should shoot for three to five minutes nonstop; advanced athletes can do five to eight minutes for starters. In many of my dance classes, we do at least fifteen minutes of nonstop abs, and many of those women have amazing abs.

Before we get rolling with the specific exercises, take a quick look at these Guidelines for Amazing Abs. Then we will get it on with the how-to instructions on my nonstop ab circuit.

- Having toned abs is a lifestyle decision. You must make the commitment to stay on the complete program that includes dance, cardio, weight training, and a healthy diet. It does not take that much time to get it right, but you have to be disciplined.
- Use a smooth, controlled motion, not a jerky movement. This workout is not a race. Use correct form and force your abs to contract without resting.
- Ab training is only one part of trimming the waistline. You need to eat a nutritious, low-fat diet (see chapter 5 for details and menu plans). Cardio is another key because it helps burn body fat and calories. Perform aerobic activity (per chapter 2 guidelines) for thirty minutes, three to five times per week. Start off slowly and work your way up until you can train at a fairly difficult level, which burns more calories than moving at a slow pace.
- Beginners should think "progressively." If you can't complete the whole workout the first time out—don't worry . . . it is not a big deal. Add one to two minutes to the workout each time you train as endurance and time allow. As you become more advanced, double the length of each exercise to reach a total of ten minutes and try to perform the more advanced exercises that really tone those abs.

- You will not see your abs until the fat is stripped away. Patience, sisters! It takes time and consistency to realize your goals. But with a sustained effort you will make it to the Promised Land.
- All the following exercises begin in the "halfway" position, which means you are in the up position, shoulders off the floor. From there, your shoulders never touch the floor until the end of the workout.
- Beginners may be tempted to allow their shoulders to touch the floor—relaxing the abdominals, but that will work against everything you are striving so hard to achieve. Keep your abs contracted the whole time, and you will look fine in no time.

Okay, let's get started.

Exercise One: Simple Crunch

TARGET AREA: UPPER ABS.

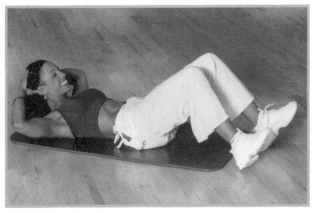

Starting position: Your heels should be on the floor with your toes point-ing up in the air. Both hands behind the head for support. Relax your head into your hands like a pillow to take the tension off the neck. Note in the photo that I'm in the halfway position, with my shoulders off the floor and my hips rotated forward.

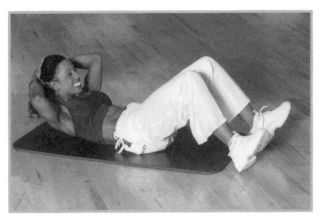

I'm contracting my abs the entire time, raising up slowly and ever so slightly, squeezing my abs at the top. Return to the start (halfway) position. Do not lie all the way back so that your shoulders are resting on the floor.

Exercise Two: Full Crunch and Simple Crunch

TARGET AREA: UPPER ABS.

Starting position: You need to have enough flexibility to lift your legs up in the air and in line with your hips. If you lack flexibility, do not perform this exercise (it puts too much strain on the lower back if you can't get into the correct position).

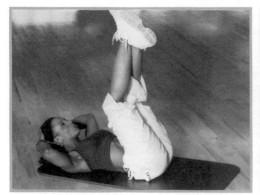 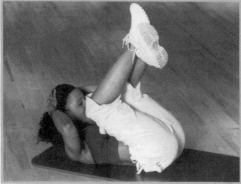

From the halfway position (meaning you're in the up position and your shoulders are off the ground) crunch in, bring your knees to your chest, and raise your chest to meet your knees. Hold for the contraction for a count of three and return to the simple crunch starting (halfway) position. Follow with a simple crunch.

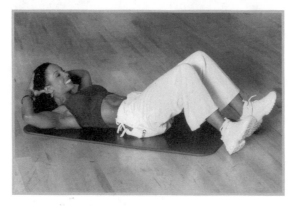

Exercise Three: Bicycle Crunch

TARGET AREAS: UPPER AND LOWER ABS.

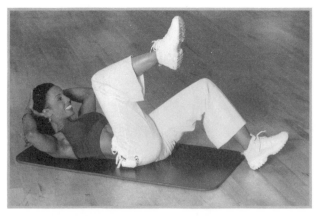

Starting position: From the halfway position, bring your right knee in to your chest as your body crunches up.

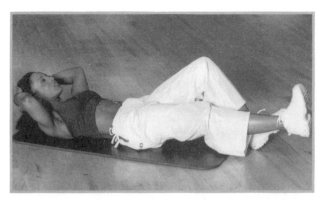

As your upper body returns to the halfway position, extend your right leg straight out, but do not let it touch the floor. Squeeze and contract the abs. You work your upper abs as you bring your knee to your chest; you target lower abs as you extend your leg and return to the halfway position. Repeat with the left leg.

Exercise Four: Oblique Crunch

TARGET AREA: OBLIQUES.

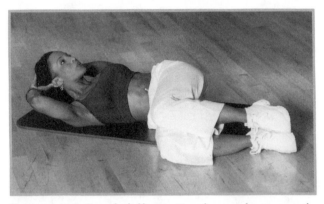

Starting position: From the halfway position, drop your knees over to the right side of your body so that you are in a twisted position. Your shoulders should stay flat; don't turn your head and neck in the direction of your lower body, as they should continue to remain in the simple crunch start position.

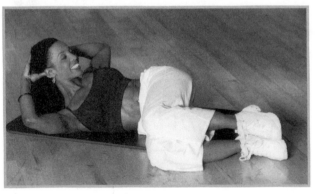

Contract the obliques by raising your torso. Repeat on the left side.

The Stretching Session in Sequence

This routine should be followed after dancing and weight training, six days per week. Always break into a sweat before you stretch. You had a complete warm-up for dance and weight-training workouts, so the stretching session makes for an excellent cooldown. Do ten reps of each stretch before moving on to the next one.

OPENING POSITION

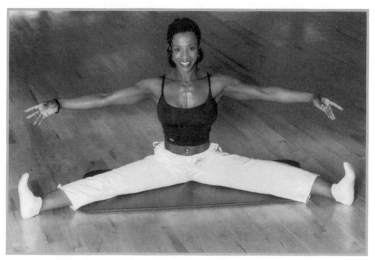

This is the opening posture of the entire stretch routine. Rest on your "sit" bones and spread your legs and arms as far apart as your range of motion and flexibility will allow.

SIDE STRETCH

Target areas: Upper body and hamstrings.

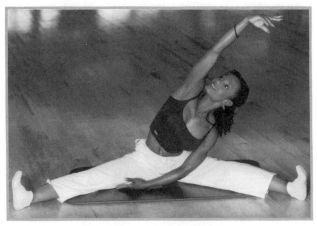

Reach your left arm over your head and lean your torso to the right, stretching the left side of your upper body and the hamstring of the right leg, which your upper body is falling toward. Hold until you feel the stretch, then release.

HEAD-TO-KNEE STRETCH

Target areas: Hamstrings and lower back.

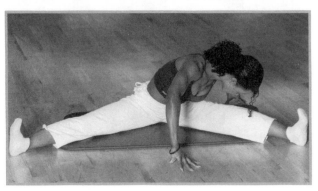

From the side stretch, turn your torso to face downward toward your leg to stretch the hamstring of your leg.

Repeat the side stretch and the head-to-knee stretch on the left side.

CENTER STRETCH

Target area: Center part of hamstrings.

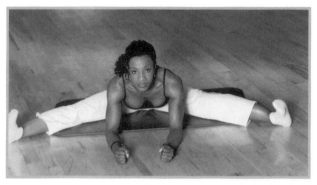

Place your elbows on the floor in front of you, shoulder-width apart, to stretch the hamstrings. Lean forward and feel the stretch. If you find this difficult, bend your knees in this spread-leg position. That will allow you to bring your upper body forward. Hold until you feel the stretch, then release.

ADVANCED CENTER STRETCH

Target area: Center part of hamstrings.

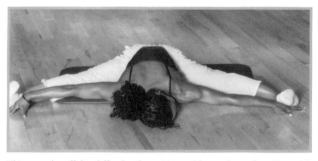

This stretch will be difficult, if not impossible, to do at first. But with enough flexibility, you can do it. From the center stretch position, bring your torso all the way forward so that your chest is lying on the floor. Spread your arms as far apart as possible to stretch the hamstrings fully. Hold until you feel the stretch, then release. Perform in addition to the center stretch to increase hamstring flexibility.

SEATED HIP AND HAMSTRING STRETCH

Target areas: Hips and hamstrings.

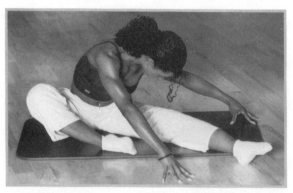

In a seated position, pull your left foot into your body, bending your knee, and stretch your right leg out at an angle from your body. Stretch your upper body over the straight leg. Hold until you feel the stretch, then release.

QUAD STRETCH

Target areas: Quads and hips.

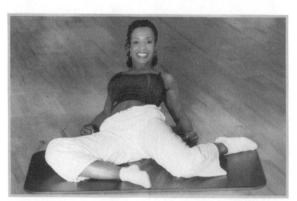

This stretch follows in sequence from the seated hip and hamstring stretch: You take the leg that was straight in the seated hip and hamstring stretch and bend it backward. Lean back and stretch the front of the thigh. Hold until you feel the stretch, then release.

Repeat the seated hip and hamstring stretch and quad stretch on the other side.

PIKE STRETCH

Target areas: Hamstrings and lower back.

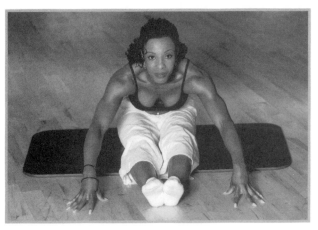

Sit on the floor with your legs outstretched straight in front of you. With your hands on the floor to the sides and in front of you, try to put your stomach and your chest on your thighs to stretch the hamstrings and lower back. Hold until you feel the stretch, then release.

ADVANCED PIKE STRETCH

Target areas: Hamstrings and lower back.

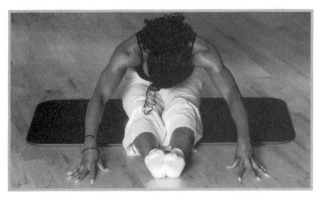

Repeat the pike stretch but complete the movement by bringing your head down as well. Hold until you feel the stretch, then release.

HIP, LOWER-BACK, AND HAMSTRING STRETCH

Target areas: All of the above.

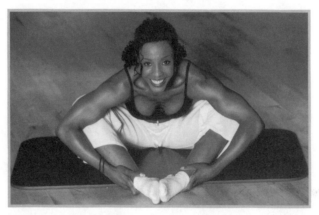

Seated on the floor, bring both feet together in front of you, not too close to your crotch, and open out your knees. Bring your stomach and chest forward to stretch your hips, lower back, and hamstrings. Hold until you feel the stretch, then release.

ADVANCED HIP, LOWER-BACK, AND HAMSTRING STRETCH

Target areas: All of the above.

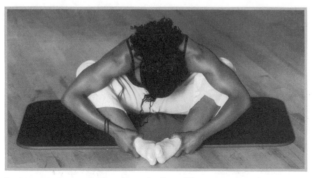

In this variation on the hip, lower-back, and hamstring stretch, you bring your head all the way down after the stomach and chest come forward. Hold until you feel the stretch, then release.

LOWER-BACK STRETCH

Target area: Lower back.

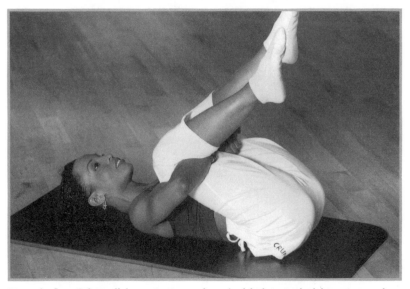

Lie on the floor. Release all the tension in your lower back by bringing both knees to your chest. Grab behind your knees and pull them as close to your chest as possible. Hold until you feel the stretch, then release.

ONE-LEG-AT-A-TIME LOWER-BACK AND HIP STRETCH
Target areas: Lower back and hips.

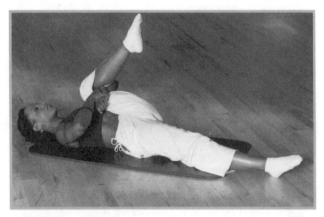

Lie on the floor with your legs stretched straight out. Bring your right knee to the right side of your chest. Hold until you feel the stretch, then release.

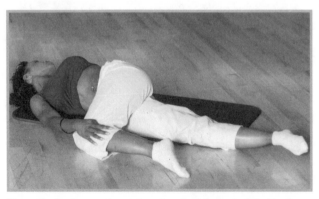

Then take that knee and push it against the floor on the left side of your body over your left leg to stretch the hip and lower back. Hold until you feel the stretch, then release. Repeat this stretch on the other side.

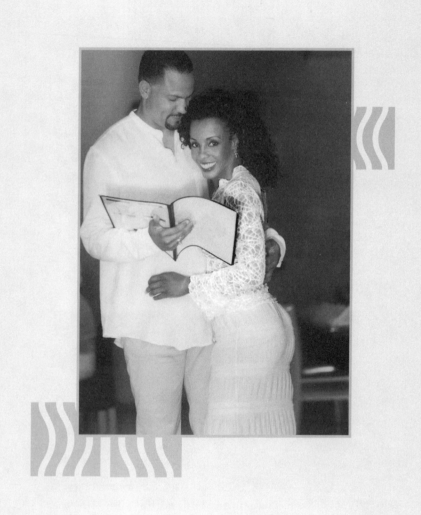

5

Ideal Nutrition for the African-American Woman on the Move

Black women are nurtured in a family environment that puts a priority on eating well. Our moms serve traditional dishes like macaroni and cheese, collard greens, fried chicken, and meatballs with spaghetti. Sunday picnics after church always include ribs, fried chicken, and corn bread.

We grow up with very specific ideas about body image (bigger is better) and portion size (bigger is better). My mom always cooked good dinners for our family, but we never ate breakfast. In fact, she would rarely eat before 3 P.M., and that example influenced how I structured my diet. On weekends she would cook pancakes and hot cereal for breakfast but during the week, we had little or no food until the afternoon. Which brings me to my first rule of eating:

Eat Breakfast—Even If You Are Not Hungry: I know the feeling of having no interest in eating after waking up in the morning. It is second nature for me to skip breakfast. But getting in the habit of eating a good breakfast will provide you with more energy throughout the day and minimize the risk of snacking on donuts or other sweets while you are at work or driving around town on business.

As you can see in the daily meal plans, you have many healthy options that will take about two to five minutes to prepare before starting your busy day. You can heat up low-fat turkey sausages, scramble egg whites (you can purchase premeasured egg whites in the dairy cases of many stores), microwave or toast frozen pancakes, sprinkle fresh fruit over low-fat yogurt, or drizzle maple syrup over hot oatmeal.

Dancers have a tendency to starve themselves to get lean, and that's a very unhealthy lifestyle. I was a dance student at NYU and a dancer and singer on Broadway, and the people I was hanging out with after college had terrible eating habits. When I started competing in aerobics events, I was exposed to fitness experts and nutritionists who turned me on to eating egg whites, grilled chicken breasts, and the other low-fat, high-protein foods associated with sports science and peak performance.

Though all these "fitness people" have influenced my perspective on diet, I'm still a sister who likes to eat the good-tasting *soul food* that is so much a part of our Afro-American culture. I'm going to share advice on cooking the traditional foods in healthy ways. You don't have to give up the foods you love to eat just because you are trying to get leaner and look and feel better.

Fried Chicken

Substitute lemon pepper for salt as a seasoning. Fry in canola or safflower oil to use healthier fat without sacrificing any flavor. Serve fresh vegetables and green salads with fat-free or low-fat salad dressing with the chicken instead of potato salad that's high in fat thanks to all that mayonnaise. If you want to serve potato salad, try substituting a little olive oil or Dijon mustard for the usual high-fat mayonnaise. Or try a low-fat variety of mayo.

If you are really trying to cut back on fat, try "oven-fried" chicken. Crumble cornflakes seasoned with lemon pepper and place in a large bowl. Whisk four egg whites and set aside in another bowl. Dip the chicken in the egg whites, roll into the crumbled cornflakes mixture, and bake at 350 degrees for thirty-five to forty minutes.

Macaroni and Cheese

My mom loves this stuff, and it always amazes me how she can eat so much of it, especially since it is usually prepared with the worst possible American cheese.

Here are three quick and easy methods of trimming the fat in mac and cheese: Use non-fat cheese (this will cut the calories by one-half and no one will ever know the difference), skim milk (instead of whole milk), and low-cal butter (instead of the real thing). Prep and cook as usual.

SPAGHETTI AND MEATBALLS

Nothing wrong with this meal, sisters. Pasta is a good source of carbohydrates that burn slow and steady over the course of your workouts. Tomato sauce is typically low in fat, but be sure to read labels to find a brand that has less than 3 grams of fat per one-half cup serving.

Meatballs are another story. The goal is portion control, and that means limiting meatballs to two per serving. If you are cooking at home, make your meatballs out of 95 percent lean ground beef to reduce the fat.

CATFISH

Instead of deep-frying the fish every time you prepare this wonderful southern specialty, try cooking the catfish (choose filets that are on the thin side) in a non-stick skillet lightly sprayed with vegetable oil. Coat with cornmeal (as per usual) and grill on both sides on a medium-high flame.

CORN BREAD

The good thing about corn bread is that it is relatively low in sugar. The bad thing about corn bread is that it is often loaded with oil, which bumps up the calorie count. When baking corn bread, it is possible to substitute unsweetened applesauce for one-half of the oil that's called for in the recipe. For example, a recipe that tells you to use one cup of oil can be changed to one-half cup of oil and one-half cup of applesauce. This will lighten up the recipe, and add a delicious new nuance to your corn bread.

CANDIED YAMS

Yams, or sweet potatoes, are a great source of energy that are rich in fiber and potassium. These slow-burning carbs will help fill you up and keep you from bingeing on potato chips, pizza, chocolate cake, and ice cream.

Avoid the "giant" yams; instead, opt for small- to medium-sized yams to keep calories under control. Top the yams with low-fat butter and a sugar substitute you can cook with instead of loading them up with real butter and honey.

GREENS

Mustard and collard greens taste great and are low in calories—unless, of course, you add bacon or salt pork. And who does not prepare greens with some pork for flavor? Try to limit the amount of bacon and experiment with turkey bacon as a low-fat alternative.

MY 30 STEPS TO A HEALTHY DIET
FOR BLACK WOMEN

1. CARBS ARE FOR ENERGY

All the dancing, cardio, and weight training I'm making you do requires carbs to fuel your workouts. Carbs are made up of chains of glucose molecules, and the body loves to absorb those sugars for energy.

2. FAVOR COMPLEX CARBS

Complex carbs—built from long chains of sugars—burn slowly to fuel those longer workouts designed to shed calories and trim the waist. Complex carbs include vegetables, fruit, oatmeal, pasta, yams, brown rice and other whole grains, and potatoes.

3. MONITOR YOUR SATURATED-FAT INTAKE

Saturated fats, common in fattier types of meat, increase the risk of cardiovascular disease and other related health problems (hypertension). Eat lean meat instead of high-fat cuts. Filet mignon, lean turkey breast, chicken breast (skinless) and whey protein powder are excellent alternative protein sources.

4. EAT HEALTHY FATS

Foods containing unsaturated fat (the good fat) with plenty of healthful Omega-3 and Omega-6 fatty acids include fish, avocados, flaxseed oil, olives, seeds, nuts, and canola and olive oils.

5. DRINK LOTS OF WATER

Sisters: This is just simple common sense. Drinking water allows nutrients to move quickly through your bloodstream and right into the muscle cells. Plus, water contains valuable minerals that aid in digestion. Drink as much water as possible—aim for at least eight 8-ounce glasses per day.

6. DON'T FORGET THE FIBER

Fiber helps to lean you out and works with protein to feed your muscles. Fruits, vegetables, and grains are the best sources of fiber in your daily diet.

7. EGGS ARE A VALUABLE SOURCE OF PROTEIN

It took some time for me to get used to eating eggs in the morning. But it is true that egg whites are a good source of low-cal, fat-free protein and the yolks do offer the benefits of other nutrients and lecithin. Try to minimize your intake of yolks, though. They are high in fat and cholesterol.

8. EAT VEGETABLES DAILY

Try to eat at least a serving of vegetables with every meal (except breakfast). Vegetables will help to keep you lean (thanks to the fiber) and easily processing all the protein in your diet.

9. Fruits Are Crucial for Women's Health

Fruit is a reliable source of carbs, fiber, and antioxidants. Eat two pieces of fruit, per serving, per day.

10. Use Protein Supplements As Needed

Most of the sisters I hang with do not like protein drinks—too much trouble to fix, and the taste is not to our liking. But the protein bars are improving, and are an easy and fast way to increase protein intake if you are too busy to eat right. Go to a health health-food store and experiment with different brands of protein bars until you find something you like. Look for protein drinks and bars low in carbohydrates (including sugar).

11. Supplement with a Multivitamin

Take a multivitamin with breakfast as an insurance policy against having a bad food day and ending up at Mickey D's or Burger King when you least expect it. Plus, the vitamin boost will contribute to your overall well-being.

12. Minerals Are Essential

Most once-per-day multivitamins are weak in the mineral department. I recommend taking extra calcium for burning fat and elevating metabolism, and magnesium for improving your dance and weight-training performance. Get your calcium from 1,000 milligrams per day of supplement-source calcium or two cups of fat-free dairy and take 450 milligrams of magnesium.

13. Vitamin C Offers Protection

This potent antioxidant protects the immune system and allows it to work more efficiently. Multivitamins contain small quantities of vitamin C, but if you want to try additional supplementation take 500 milligrams per day.

14. Vitamin E Equals Preservation

Vitamin E preserves and prolongs the life of red blood cells and helps to promote the uptake of oxygen by the muscles. About 400 International Units daily (including the amount in your multivitamin) is enough to get it done.

15. Eat a Small Meal before Training

I know many dancers who never eat so much as a crumb before rehearsals, but it is healthier to eat a small meal (about 200 calories) to energize your training without making you too full.

16. Eat Protein at Every Meal

The goal is to prevent your body from burning muscle tissue as fuel during your busy workout schedule. Eating protein at every meal ensures that your muscles will burn protein—not your valuable tissue—to sustain the intensity of your workouts.

17. Take in a Big Meal Just After an Intense Workout

Eat a big meal—ideally one from the "Dinner" section in the 7-Day Meal Plan—after training to help promote recovery and stimulate fast results.

18. Cut Back on Carbs at Night

Strive to take in more carbs early in the day and before and after training. You have less use for energy-yielding calories right before you go to bed. And if your body can't use them, it stores them as fat.

19. Avoid Junk Food

I know how the game is played: You are over at a girlfriend's house after work and she has a big plate of potato chips and Cheetos on the coffee table. What are you going to do? Don't eat the junk food! Always hold out for raw vegetables and fruit in social situations. Stay away from baked goods made with white flour (cake, cookies, and donuts!) and minimize contact with processed meats and the drive-thru at McDonald's.

20. Cheat-Meals Once a Week Are Cool

Hey, I'm not trying to take all the fun out of your diet. I want you to look and feel better, and that requires self-sacrifice and self-control. If you must eat a donut, go ahead and enjoy. Just don't make a habit of cheating on your diet. One cheat-meal per week is about right for the body and mind.

21. Pay Attention to What Your Body Tells You

All the meal plans in this chapter have been tested by a nutritionist, but that does not mean that every sister is going to react the same way to each food item. Figure out what works best for you and trust what your body tells you about what to eat and what to avoid on a daily basis.

22. Read Labels

Pay attention to the number of servings per package and how all the nutritional info adds up. Do the math! Look for sugar content. If sugar, sucrose, glucose, or fructose is one of the first items on the ingredient list on the package, put that product right back on the shelf.

23. Trim All Visible Fat from Meat

It would be nice to be able to eat filet mignon all the time, but it is kind of expensive. When you must buy the less expensive cuts of beef, always trim the fat carefully.

24. Baking Is Better

Instead of frying your foods, try baking them. You need to do this in a preheated oven to allow the heat to seal in the juices. With low-fat baking, use a nonstick pan or a pan lightly sprayed with vegetable oil.

25. Grilling Is Hot

I enjoy grilling meats and vegetables because it seals in the flavors with dry heat. I always use a nonstick grill and make sure it is hot enough before I start to cook.

26. Roasting Is Right On

Once again, this cooking method relies on dry heat to seal in flavor. I will roast on the rack of a preheated oven or in a roasting pan.

27. Think Before You Order in a Restaurant

Eating out is the toughest part of staying on course with the plan of action. Order your meats broiled or grilled instead of fried. Stay away from french fries and order a side of fresh fruit or steamed vegetables. Chicken and fish are leaner than red meat, though a lean steak like a filet mignon is okay. If you opt for the salad, make sure you choose a low-fat dressing and avoid all the fatty toppings—cheeses, eggs, ham, bacon bits, oily croutons. By the time all of these extras are piled on, a salad can be as fattening as a cheeseburger. Limit dairy and don't go crazy with a big dessert—unless, of course, it is a special occasion and you are counting this as your cheat-meal.

28. Limit Sodium Intake

Sodium chloride (salt) often causes bloating and raises blood pressure. Try lemon pepper instead of table salt (as in the fried-chicken recipe) or use a salt substitute, which is a blend of regular table salt and potassium chloride (which lowers rather than raises blood pressure).

29. Use Spices to Make Food Fun

When you cut the fat—not to mention the salt—from dishes, sometimes flavor is sacrificed. Salsa, Tabasco sauce, paprika, fresh sage, and dill are all useful additions to make bland foods taste better. Be creative. Don't be afraid to experiment with new tastes and textures.

30. Don't Look for Shortcuts

It is always tempting to say "Forget it" and to look for a quick-fix way to lose weight. You'll never find that magic bullet, girlfriend. The only real way to design that dream body with the slim waist, rounded butt, and toned muscles is to take the whole diet trip. There are no shortcuts to success!

THE WORK IT OUT 7-DAY MEAL PLAN

Note: This is not a plan that is written in stone and has to be followed to the letter. Pick and choose what you like. Substitute freely and experiment with different food combinations. I have tried to include all the foods that you like, but in moderation and prepared in a healthy way to offer a best-of-both-worlds approach: The goal is to eat healthy and to eat well.

DAY 1*

Breakfast

	CALORIES	CARBOHYDRATES (GR)	PROTEIN (GR)	FAT (GR)
1 turkey sausage link	157	2	17	9
2 egg whites	30	0	6	0
1 cup shredded potatoes, grilled	153	32	4	1

Snack

	CALORIES	CARBOHYDRATES (GR)	PROTEIN (GR)	FAT (GR)
2 cups strawberries	90	21	2	1

Lunch

	CALORIES	CARBOHYDRATES (GR)	PROTEIN (GR)	FAT (GR)
Lean Cuisine: Spaghetti & Meatballs	290	36	20	7
1 large green salad with a fat-free dressing	50	11	1	0

*All nutrition data compiled by Chris Aceto.

DAY 1 *(continued)*

Snack

	CALORIES	CARBOHYDRATES (GR)	PROTEIN (GR)	FAT (GR)
1 cup fruit cocktail (in juice)	120	30	1	0

Dinner

	CALORIES	CARBOHYDRATES (GR)	PROTEIN (GR)	FAT (GR)
4 ounces marinated steak, grilled	268	0	31	14
1 medium yam, baked (6 ounces) with 2 teaspoons whipped low-fat butter	288	46	3	10
1 cup collard greens	40	4	4	1

DAY 2

Breakfast

	Calories	Carbohydrates (gr)	Protein (gr)	Fat (gr)
2 pancakes (buy frozen; cook in microwave or toaster)	120	34	3	2
1 banana, sliced	100	24	0	0
8 ounces fat-free vanilla yogurt (add fruit for flavor)	110	17	8	0

Snack

	Calories	Carbohydrates (gr)	Protein (gr)	Fat (gr)
2 Fig Newton bars	80	19	0	1

Lunch

	Calories	Carbohydrates (gr)	Protein (gr)	Fat (gr)
1 medium catfish	223	0	22	11
1 cup rice	200	44	5	1
½ cup black beans	80	12	7	1

DAY 2 (continued)

Lunch (continued)

	CALORIES	CARBOHYDRATES (GR)	PROTEIN (GR)	FAT (GR)
1 medium portion mixed vegetables	45	12	1	0

Snack

	CALORIES	CARBOHYDRATES (GR)	PROTEIN (GR)	FAT (GR)
½ bagel	100	23	2	1
with 3 table-spoons fat-free cream cheese	80	5	14	0

Dinner

	CALORIES	CARBOHYDRATES (GR)	PROTEIN (GR)	FAT (GR)
Meat loaf (made with lean ground beef)	223	5	24	8
1 cup mashed potatoes	204	40	2	4
¾ cup peas	90	15	5	0

DAY 3

Breakfast

	CALORIES	CARBOHYDRATES (GR)	PROTEIN (GR)	FAT (GR)
½ cup (dry-measure) oatmeal	200	27	7	3
⅔ cup fat-free vanilla yogurt	72	11	6	0
2 tablespoons raisins	84	20	1	0

Snack

1 slice low-fat corn bread	196	38	2	4

Lunch

2 slices whole-wheat bread	140	28	6	2
3 slices ham	135	0	12	10
1 slice fat-free cheese	35	2	5	0
1 tablespoon mustard	10	1	1	0

DAY 3 *(continued)*

Lunch *(continued)*

	CALORIES	CARBOHYDRATES (GR)	PROTEIN (GR)	FAT (GR)
1 medium portion mixed vegetables	45	12	1	0

Snack

1 slice watermelon	102	23	2	1

Dinner

Healthy Choice: Shrimp Marinara	260	51	10	1
1 medium portion mixed vegetables	45	12	1	0

DAY 4

Breakfast

	CALORIES	CARBOHYDRATES (GR)	PROTEIN (GR)	FAT (GR)
3 egg whites	45	0	9	0
2 slices whole-wheat toast	140	28	6	2
4 teaspoons low-sugar jam	60	15	0	0

Snack

1 low-fat bran muffin	217	39	4	5

Lunch

1 serving macaroni and cheese	350	36	11	17
1 medium portion mixed vegetables	45	12	1	0

DAY 4 *(continued)*

Snack

	CALORIES	CARBOHYDRATES (GR)	PROTEIN (GR)	FAT (GR)
10 apple-flavored rice cakes (mini)	100	18	2	0

Dinner

6 pieces sushi	450	61	24	12
1 large green salad	50	11	1	0

DAY 5

Breakfast

	CALORIES	CARBOHYDRATES (GR)	PROTEIN (GR)	FAT (GR)
½ bagel	100	23	2	1
3 egg whites	45	0	9	0
8-ounce glass of orange juice	80	20	0	0

Snack

8 ounces fat-free yogurt	110	17	8	0

Lunch

1 small pita bread	128	23	5	0
3 slices turkey	85	0	15	3
2 tablespoons fat-free mayo	30	7	0	0
1 small apple	80	20	0	0

DAY 5 *(continued)*

Snack

	CALORIES	CARBOHYDRATES (GR)	PROTEIN (GR)	FAT (GR)
3 rice cakes	210	21	1	0
2 slices fat-free cheese	105	6	15	0

Dinner

	CALORIES	CARBOHYDRATES (GR)	PROTEIN (GR)	FAT (GR)
1 small (single-serving) cheese pizza	354	54	12	9
1 large salad	50	11	1	0
Low-fat dressing	80	0	2	8

DAY 6

Breakfast

	CALORIES	CARBOHYDRATES (GR)	PROTEIN (GR)	FAT (GR)
2 slices whole-wheat toast	140	26	5	2
3 egg whites	45	0	9	0
3 teaspoons low-sugar jam	60	15	0	0

Snack

	CALORIES	CARBOHYDRATES (GR)	PROTEIN (GR)	FAT (GR)
8 ounces fat-free yogurt	110	17	8	0

Lunch

	CALORIES	CARBOHYDRATES (GR)	PROTEIN (GR)	FAT (GR)
1 cup rice	200	45	5	1
3 ounces lean ground beef	123	0	15	9
⅓ cup salsa	30	7	0	0

DAY 6 *(continued)*

Snack

	CALORIES	CARBOHYDRATES (GR)	PROTEIN (GR)	FAT (GR)
Banana	100	24	0	0

Dinner

	CALORIES	CARBOHYDRATES (GR)	PROTEIN (GR)	FAT (GR)
Fast-food grilled chicken sandwich	294	35	25	6
Diet Coke	0	0	0	0
1 large green salad	50	11	1	0

DAY 7

Breakfast

	CALORIES	CARBOHYDRATES (GR)	PROTEIN (GR)	FAT (GR)
1 piece low-fat corn bread	130	26	3	1–3
3 egg whites with 1 slice fat-free cheese	80	0	9	0
1 cup melon	70	16	0	0

Snack

	CALORIES	CARBOHYDRATES (GR)	PROTEIN (GR)	FAT (GR)
1 piece fruit	100–165	25–40	1-3	0–4

Lunch

	CALORIES	CARBOHYDRATES (GR)	PROTEIN (GR)	FAT (GR)
1 cup pasta with 2 meatballs	385	59	16	8
1 medium portion mixed vegetables	45	12	1	0

DAY 7 *(continued)*

Snack

	CALORIES	CARBOHYDRATES (GR)	PROTEIN (GR)	FAT (GR)
2 cups air-popped popcorn	100	24	1	0

Dinner

1 piece fried chicken	320	6	23	14
1 garden salad with low-fat dressing	100	6	0	5
1 small yam with low-fat butter	230	37	5	7

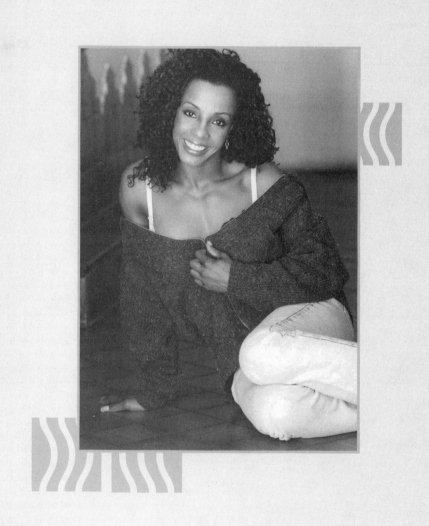

6

Success Stories and Parting Words

I'll leave you with great hope for the future of black women in our culture. I want to tell you about two strong sisters who have used this program to change their lives, lose weight, and improve the quality of their health and the level of their self-confidence.

Lord knows we have our work cut out for us when it comes to changing the long-term health trends for sisters in the United States. Remember the statistics on women's health in the black community in the Introduction? But it can be done with a little hard work and determination. And I know you're determined; otherwise you wouldn't have bought this book.

Let me tell you about two friends of mine who have lost weight and improved their life through exercise, proper nutrition, and a steady regimen of dancing to shake it all up.

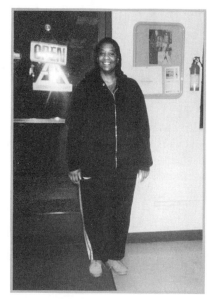

(Before)

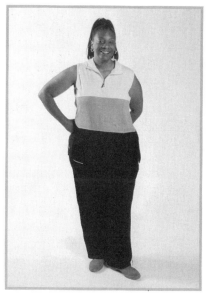

(After)

FRANÇOISE BROUSSARD

OCCUPATION: *Advertising Department*, Premiere *magazine*

HEALTH CONCERN: *Overweight/obesity*

AMOUNT OF WEIGHT LOST: *31 pounds in less than three months*

I met MaDonna three years ago at a fitness seminar in Pasadena, where she was teaching a cardio dance class. I had dabbled in dance classes for several years but was never able to be consistent about my fitness routine. Once I met MaDonna, my life changed right away. She is such a great teacher, motivator, and fitness expert that I could not help but get hooked on her classes and her system. No matter how busy I am with my job, I always drive to her classes—whether it is at Sports Club/LA or Crunch in West Hollywood. The dance workout helps me burn fat and gives me something to look forward to all day at the office. That extrinsic motivation helps me perform at a higher level. The nutrition advice is what has really pushed me into losing weight and feeling healthier and happier. MaDonna's program works because she cares about her students and wants all women to lead healthier and happier lives.

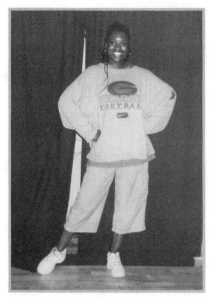

(Before)

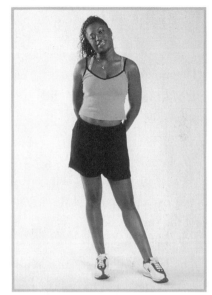

(After)

KEJO THOMAS

OCCUPATION: *Student*

HEALTH CONCERN: *Hypertension/weight loss*

AMOUNT OF WEIGHT LOST: *15 pounds in four months*

I've taken MaDonna's classes for more than five years, and no matter where she goes to teach, I follow in pursuit of the best hip-hop teacher I've ever met in my life. I know that I would be overweight if MaDonna was not right there to keep it real for me and to make sure that I was being consistent with every facet of my program: dance, weight training, cardio, and diet. The diet part is the hardest—I know most sisters don't want to give up the cheesecake and the banana pudding and all that good food we grew up with. But MaDonna has taught me to pay attention to what I'm eating and the connection between eating well and feeling well. Thanks to MaDonna, I'm on the road to health and having a great body.

PARTING WORDS FROM YOUR "TEACHER"

The program I've created is for *all women*. When you look at Françoise and Kejo, you are looking at real people—they are not skinny or ripped like fitness girls. But they are consistent, constantly improving, and totally committed to getting better and better each and every day.

Françoise still has a way to go, but the beautiful thing is that she has lost thirty pounds in a matter of weeks. Her setbacks in the past occurred because she was not consistent when it came to eating well and following all the elements of any given program. She found the elements of the Work It Out program fun and easy to follow and has been able to stick to it, with great results.

Kejo has been able to keep her weight down by attending dance classes consistently, though she has the propensity to gain weight easily without regular exercise. She is happy when she dances and frustrated when she does not find the time to do so.

The key to making this program fly is finding out what you like to do and matching that up against what you have to do. Follow the meal plans but be flexible, show yourself some forgiveness, and have a scoop of ice cream for your soul. Dance to your heart's content, lift weights to ensure the health of your bones, and ride the bike or run on the treadmill to minimize the risk of coronary heart disease and obesity.

Sisters are doing it for themselves. But we still have to keep the faith and live the life that brings emotional well-being, spiritual fulfillment, and a healthy, sexy body to be proud of.

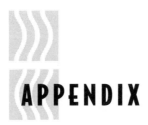

APPENDIX

THE COMPLETE "WORK IT OUT" WEEKLY SCHEDULE

MONDAY

30 minutes of cardio (either treadmill or stationary bike) at 55 to 85% of your max heart rate.

Lower-Body Weight Training (20–30 minutes)

Dumbbell squats = 4 sets of 12 reps
Leg extensions = 4 sets of 15 reps
Leg curls = 4 sets of 15 reps
Dumbbell lunges = 4 sets of 15 reps

Post-workout stretching (5–10 minutes)
Abdominal circuit (5–10 minutes)

TUESDAY

Dance Class #1: *Dance Street*
5-minute dance warm-up

Appendix

5-minute dance stretch—standing lunges, lower-back stretches, head circles
30 minutes of "Dance Street"

Post-workout stretching (5–10 minutes)
Abdominal circuit (5–10 minutes)

WEDNESDAY

30 minutes of cardio (either treadmill or stationary bike) at 55 to 85% of max heart rate.

Upper-Body Weight Training (30 minutes)

Wide-grip pulldowns = 2–4 sets of 10–15 reps
One-arm dumbbell rows = 2–4 sets of 10–15 reps
Dumbbell flat bench presses = 2–4 sets of 10–15 reps
Incline dumbbell flyers = 2–4 sets of 10–15 reps
Triceps pressdowns = 2–3 sets of 10–15 reps or
Triceps kickbacks = 3 sets of 10–15 reps
Standing dumbbell curls = 2–3 sets of 10–15 reps *or*
Hammer curls = 2–3 sets of 10–15 reps
Dumbbell shoulder presses = 2–3 sets of 10–15 reps *or*
Front raises = 2–3 sets of 10–15 reps
Standing lateral raises = 2–3 sets of 10–12 reps

Post-workout stretching (5–10 minutes)
Post-workout abdominal circuit (5–10 minutes)

THURSDAY

Dance Class #2: *Afro-Latino*

5 minute dance warm-up
5-minute dance stretch—standing lunges, lower-back stretches, head circles

30 minutes of "Afro-Latino"
Post-workout stretching (5–10 minutes)
Abdominal circuit (5–10 minutes)

FRIDAY

Repeat Monday's workout.

SATURDAY

Dance Class #3: *Cardio Dance*

5-minute dance warm-up
5-minute dance stretch—standing lunges, lower-back stretches, head circles
30 minutes of "Cardio Dance"

Post-workout stretching (5–10 minutes)
Abdominal circuit (5–10 minutes)

SUNDAY

Rest.

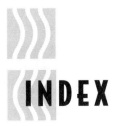

INDEX

Index

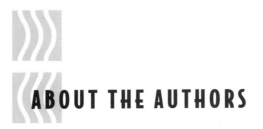

ABOUT THE AUTHORS

MaDonna Grimes holds a B.S. in Dance Education from Ohio State University, where she studied classical dance. She earned a master's degree in Dance Performance and Choreography from New York University. Her many professional achievements include winning titles in dance (USA Dance Champion), aerobics (USA Aerobics Champion), and fitness (she was the first black woman to receive both the Miss Fitness America and the Miss Fitness International titles); founding, directing, and coordinating the MaDonna Grimes Fitness & Dance Theatre Company in Los Angeles and owning the Athletic Garage, a dance and fitness studio in Pasadena, California; and working as creative director for various health clubs, including Bally's, Sports Club/LA, and Gold's Gym. She also has a line of dance videos—*I Just Wanna Dance*, levels 1, 2, and 3. MaDonna is a professional dancer and choreographer with an international following in the hip-hop and fitness industry. She lives in Los Angeles, California. Visit her website at www.madonna-grimes.com.

Jim Rosenthal has worked in journalism for the past twenty years. He is currently a senior writer and women's training editor for Weider Publications, specifically, *Flex* and *Muscle & Fitness*. He is also the coauthor of seven sports/fitness books, including *Randy Johnson's Power Pitching*, *Nolan Ryan's Pitcher's Bible*, *Tony Gwynn's Total Baseball Player*, and *Kiana's Body Sculpting*. A graduate of Northwestern University in Evanston, Illinois, he lives in the Los Angeles area.